Diabetes Mellitus

Issues for the Indian Woman

Diabetes Mellitus
Issues for the Indian Woman

Editor

Sarita Bajaj MD DM (Endo, AIIMS)
FRCP (Glasgow, Edinburgh, London)
Consultant Endocrinologist
Director-Professor and Head
Department of Medicine
Moti Lal Nehru Medical College
Allahabad, Uttar Pradesh, India

Foreword

Soumya Swaminathan

JAYPEE The Health Sciences Publisher
New Delhi | London | Panama

Jaypee Brothers Medical Publishers (P) Ltd

Headquarters

Jaypee Brothers Medical Publishers (P) Ltd
4838/24, Ansari Road, Daryaganj
New Delhi 110 002, India
Phone: +91-11-43574357
Fax: +91-11-43574314
Email: jaypee@jaypeebrothers.com

Overseas Offices

J.P. Medical Ltd
83 Victoria Street, London
SW1H 0HW (UK)
Phone: +44 20 3170 8910
Fax: +44 (0)20 3008 6180
Email: info@jpmedpub.com

Jaypee-Highlights Medical Publishers Inc
City of Knowledge, Bld. 237, Clayton
Panama City, Panama
Phone: +1 507-301-0496
Fax: +1 507-301-0499
Email: cservice@jphmedical.com

Jaypee Brothers Medical Publishers (P) Ltd
17/1-B Babar Road, Block-B, Shaymali
Mohammadpur, Dhaka-1207
Bangladesh
Mobile: +08801912003485
Email: jaypeedhaka@gmail.com

Jaypee Brothers Medical Publishers (P) Ltd
Bhotahity, Kathmandu
Nepal
Phone: +977-9741283608
Email: kathmandu@jaypeebrothers.com

Website: www.jaypeebrothers.com
Website: www.jaypeedigital.com

Diabetes Mellitus: Issues for the Indian Woman / *Sarita Bajaj*

First Edition: **2018**

ISBN: 978-93-5270-259-6

Printed at: Samrat Offset Pvt. Ltd.

Dedication

I dedicate this book to the "Pretty Women" in my life:
Prem Mohini, Nehanjali, Nishika, Nyra and Yana

Contributors

EDITOR

Sarita Bajaj MD DM (Endo, AIIMS) FRCP (Glasgow, Edinburgh, London)
Consultant Endocrinologist
Director-Professor and Head
Department of Medicine
Moti Lal Nehru Medical College
Allahabad, Uttar Pradesh, India

CONTRIBUTING AUTHORS

Sanjay Agarwal MD
Director
Department of Diabetes
Aegle Clinic
Pune, Maharashtra, India

Sameer Aggarwal MD DM
Professor and Head Unit VII
Department of Medicine
Pandit Bhagwat Dayal Sharma Post Graduate Institute of Medical Sciences
Rohtak, Haryana, India

Kamlesh Ahuja DGO DNB
Consultant
Department of Obstetrics and Gynecology
Arpan Hospital
Sri Ganganagar, Rajasthan, India

Ranjit M Anjana MD Dip Diab PhD FACP FRCP (Glasgow, Edinburgh, London) FICP
Managing Director and Consultant
Department of Diabetology
Dr Mohan's Diabetes Specialities Centre
Chennai, Tamil Nadu, India

SR Aravind DNB FRCP (Glasgow and Edinburgh) FDRC DHA FRSSDI
Director
Diacon Hospital
Consultant Diabetologist
Columbia Asia Hospital
Bengaluru, Karnatkaka, India

Yatan PS Balhara MD DNB MNAMS MSc
Associate Professor
Department of Psychiatry and National Drug Dependence Treatment Centre
All India Institute of Medical Sciences
New Delhi, India

Beena Bansal MD DM
Associate Director
Department of Endocrinology and Diabetes
Medanta - The Medicity
Gurgaon, Haryana, India

Manash P Baruah MBBS MD DM FACE
Consultant and Director
Excel Care Hospital
Guwahati, Assam, India

Shweta Bhandari MD DM
Senior Resident
Department of Endocrinology and Metabolism
Institute of Medical Sciences
Varanasi, Uttar Pradesh, India

Anjali A Bhatt MD PDFD Msc
Consultant
Department of Endocrinology
Chellaram Diabetes Institute
Pune, Maharashtra, India

Aastha Chawla
MD Resident
Department of Skin
Sardar Patel Medical College
Bikaner, Rajasthan, India

Rajeev Chawla MD FRSSDI FRCP FACE
Senior Consultant and Director
North Delhi Diabetes Centre
New Delhi, India

Mala Dharmalingam MD DM
Professor and Head
Department of Endocrinology
Ramaiah Medical College
Bengaluru, Karnataka, India

Atul Dhingra MD DM
Consultant
Department of Endocrinology
Gangaram Bansal Superspeciality Hospital
Sri Ganganagar, Rajasthan, India

Mudita Dhingra MD FIAP
Consultant
Department of Pediatrics
Radhakishan Hospital
Kurukshetra, Haryana, India

Deep Dutta MD DM DNB MNAMS
Consultant and Head
Department of Endocrinology, Diabetology and Metabolic Disorders
Venkateshwar Hospital
New Delhi, India

Ipsita Ghosh MD
Senior Resident
Department of Endocrinology
Institute of Post Graduate Medical Education and Research
Kolkata, West Bengal, India

Sujoy Ghosh DM
FRCP (London, Glasgow, Edinburgh) FACE
Associate Professor
Department of Endocrinology
Institute of Post Graduate Medical Education and Research
Kolkata, West Bengal, India

Balram Gupta MSc
Research Scholar
Department of Endocrinology and Metabolism
Institute of Medical Sciences
Varanasi, Uttar Pradesh, India

Rajat Gupta MD DM
Consultant
Department of Endocrinology
Alchemist Hospital
Panchkula, Haryana, Delhi

Sunil Gupta MD FRCP (Edinburgh, Glasgow)
FACP FICP FIAMS FIACM
Deputy Managing Director
Sunil's Diabetes Care n' Research Centre
Nagpur, Maharashtra, India

Shalini Jaggi Dip Diab Dip Endo F Diab
FRSSDI FRCP (Glasgow, Edinburgh)
Consultant and Head
Department of Diabetes
Dr Mohans' Diabetes Specialities Centre
New Delhi, India

Viveka P Jyotsna DM
Professor
Department of Endocrinology and Metabolism
All India Institute of Medical Sciences
New Delhi, India

Sanjay Kalra DM
Consultant
Department of Endocrinology
Bharti Hospital
Karnal, Haryana, India

Bharti Kalra MD
Consultant
Department of Gynecology
Bharti Hospital
Karnal, Haryana, India

Parjeet Kaur MD DM
Consultant
Department of Endocrinology and Diabetes
Medanta - The Medicity
Gurgaon, Haryana, India

Deepak Khandelwal MD DM
Senior Consultant
Department of Endocrinology and Diabetes
Maharaja Agrasen Hospital
New Delhi, India

KVS Hari Kumar MD DNB
Professor
Department of Endocrinology
Army Hospital (Research and Referral)
New Delhi, India

P Venu Madhavi MD
Senior Resident
Department of Endocrinology
Osmania Medical College
Hyderabad, Telangana, India

Anuj Maheshwari MD FICP FIACM FACP FACE FRCP
Professor and Head
Department of General Medicine
Babu Banarasi Das University
Lucknow, Uttar Pradesh, India

Brij M Makkar MD FIAMS FICP FRCP FACP FACE FRSSDI
Physician
Department of Diabetes and Obesity
Diabetes and Obesity Centre
New Delhi, India

Arghya Pal MD
Consultant
Antara Psychiatric Hospital
Kolkata, West Bengal, India

Jayanta K Panda MBBS MD FACP FICP
Associate Professor
PG Department of Medicine
Shri Ramachandra Bhanj Medical College
Cuttack, Odisha, India

Madhusmita Patnaik MD
Assistant Professor
PG Department of Medicine
Shri Ramachandra Bhanj Medical College
Cuttack, Odisha, India

Gagan Priya MD DM
Senior Consultant
Department of Endocrinology
Fortis Hospital
Chandigarh, India

Nishant Raizada DM
Assistant Professor
Department of Endocrinology and Metabolism
All India Institute of Medical Sciences
New Delhi, India

Anitha Rani MSc MPhil PhD
Post Doctoral Research Fellow
Kidney Department
Prof M Viswanathan Diabetes Research Centre
Chennai, Tamil Nadu, India

Banshi Saboo MD PhD
Diabetologist
Department of Endocrinology
DIACARE
Ahmedabad, Gujarat, India

Rakesh K Sahay MD DM FACE FICP FRSSDI
Professor and Head
Department of Endocrinology
Osmania Medical College
Hyderabad, Telangana, India

Ranabir Salam MD DM FACE
Associate Professor
Department of General Medicine
Regional Institute of
Medical Sciences
Imphal, Manipur, India

Chitra Selvan DM MRCP
Assistant Professor
Department of Endocrinology
Ramaiah Medical College
Bengaluru, Karnataka, India

Shruti V Sheth MBBS
Diabetologist
Aegle Clinic
Pune, Maharashtra, India

Surya K Singh MD DM
Professor
Department of Endocrinology and Metabolism
Institute of Medical Sciences
Varanasi, Uttar Pradesh, India

Anshul Singh MD
Assistant Professor
Department of Radiotherapy and Oncology
Kasturba Medical College
Manipal, Karnataka, India

Sweta Singla MD DM
Consultant
Department of Neurology
Kalpavriksh Superspeciality Center
New Delhi, India

Usha Sriram MBBS AB Internal Medicine, Endocrinology, Diabetes and Metabolism
Director
Aceer Health
Chennai, Tamil Nadu, India

Alankar Tiwari MD
Senior Resident
Department of Gastroenterology
Moti Lal Nehru Medical College
Allahabad, Uttar Pradesh, India

AG Unnikrishnan MD DM DNB NMAMS
CEO and Chief Endocrinologist
Department of Endocrinology
Chellaram Diabetes Institute
Pune, Maharashtra, India

Ranjit Unnikrishnan MD Dip Diab FRCP (Glasgow, Edinburgh, London) FACP
Vice Chairman and Consultant
Department of Diabetology
Dr Mohan's Diabetes Specialities Centre
Chennai, Tamil Nadu, India

Sudha Vidyasagar MD
Professor
Department of Medicine
Kasturba Medical College
Manipal, Karnataka, India

Vijay Viswanathan MD PhD FICP FRCP (London, Glasgow)
Head and Chief Diabetologist
MV Hospital for Diabetes
Chennai, Tamil Nadu, India

Ganavi YP MD
Senior Resident
Department of Endocrinology
Ramaiah Medical College
Bengaluru, Karnatkaka, India

Foreword

सत्यमेव जयते
डा. सौम्या स्वामीनाथन
एमडी, एफएएससी, एफएनएएससी, एफएएमएस
सचिव, भारत सरकार
स्वास्थ्य अनुसंधान विभाग
स्वास्थ्य एवं परिवार कल्याण मंत्रालय
एवं
महानिदेशक, आई सी एम आर
Dr. Soumya Swaminathan
MD, FASc, FNASc, FAMS
Secretary to the Government of India
Department of Health Research
Ministry of Health & Family Welfare
&
Director-General, ICMR

भारतीय आयुर्विज्ञान अनुसंधान परिषद
स्वास्थ्य अनुसंधान विभाग
स्वास्थ्य एवं परिवार कल्याण मंत्रालय
वी. रामलिंगस्वामी भवन, अंसारी नगर
नई दिल्ली-110 029 (भारत)
Indian Council of Medical Research
Department of Health Research
Ministry of Health & Family Welfare
V. Ramalingaswami Bhawan, Ansari Nagar
New Delhi-110 029 (INDIA)

Soumya Swaminathan MD FASc FNASc FAMS
Secretary to the Government of India
Department of Health Research
Ministry of Health and Family Welfare
Director-General, Indian Council of Medical Research
New Delhi, India

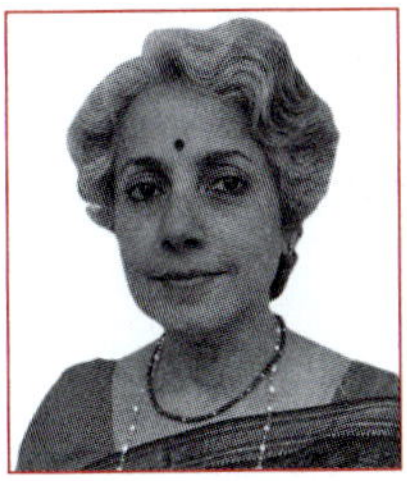

It is a great pleasure for me to write a foreword for *Diabetes Mellitus: Issues for the Indian Woman*, which is a labor of dedication and commitment by India's leading endocrine and medical specialists who have devoted their talents to highlight the importance of diabetes in women in India. It becomes very much more meaningful because the International Diabetes Federation has announced that the theme of World Diabetes Day 2017 will be "Women and Diabetes - Our Right to a Healthy Future."

The editor and contributors of this monograph have been carefully chosen to reflect expertise and established credibility in the areas that they have been assigned. The choice of topics has been well made; a synthesis of clinical and basic science and other topics that both educate and enlighten.

Despite massive explosion of online information, a monograph that has been carefully vetted by experts becomes indispensable. The lucid comprehensive and cohesive chapters are well reviewed and makes it a pleasurable reading. The book would certainly be a welcome addition to personal libraries and bookshelves.

This is a fascinating extension to the literature on diabetes.

Soumya

Soumya Swaminathan

Preface

While there are many books on the subject of women's health, in my experience, very few of them are truly created with the working primary care physician in mind. Therefore, while this book is written by leading endocrine and medical specialists, I have taken pains to design the book to be understandable by academicians and students alike; to keep abreast of rapidly changing scientific foundations, clinical research, result, and evidence-based medical practice.

Diabetes Mellitus: Issues for the Indian Woman is designed to be current, compact, and used as a clinician's handbook rather than a reference textbook. The authors have sought to provide a clear and concise guide to an optimal treatment approach. This becomes even more meaningful in context of the International Diabetes Federation having announced that the theme of World Diabetes Day 2017 will be "Women and Diabetes - Our Right to a Healthy Future."

The book is divided into seven sections and 27 chapters arranging closely related subjects into clusters. It gives an overview of women specific issues in diabetes to guidelines with chapters focusing on metabolic, endocrine, psycho-social, obstetric, and gynecologic health, comorbidities, and management.

Publishing is in every way a collaborative effort. My utmost thanks to Research Society for the Study of Diabetes in India (RSSDI) for entrusting me with this responsibility. I was fortunate to have assembled an outstanding group of authors, all recognized as leaders in their field. I thank all of them for having contributed to this book with their insightful advice and exemplary scholarship as well as for their considerable time, effort, and commitment. I am particularly grateful to Dr Sanjay Kalra for his skilful literary editing and tremendous support.

I would also like to thank Ms Barkha Arora, Editorial Coordinator at Jaypee Brothers Medical Publishers (P) Ltd., for her ready availability and unyielding patience. Her remarkable attention to detail and her pursuit of excellence have had a major impact on the book. The book could not have been edited without the dedicated help of Dr Neeraj Choudhary, Senior Acquisition Editor; Mr Gladden Saveio, Associate Editor; Dr Swati Mishra, Associate Medical Editor; and Mr Birendra Kumar, DTP Operator at Jaypee Brothers Medical Publishers (P) Ltd.

Sarita Bajaj

Contents

SECTION 1: INTRODUCTION

1. **The Guidelines: Noesis and Hopes** 1
   Sarita Bajaj, Alankar Tiwari
2. **Women Hold Up Half the Sky and More** 9
   Bharti Kalra, Sanjay Kalra
3. **Overview of Women Specific Issues in Diabetes** 12
   Atul Dhingra, Kamlesh Ahuja

SECTION 2: GLYCEMIC MANAGEMENT

4. **Lifestyle Management** 19
   Ranjit M Anjana, Ranjit Unnikrishnan
5. **Antidiabetic Drugs in Type 2 Diabetes Mellitus in Women** 25
   Ipsita Ghosh, Sarita Bajaj, Sujoy Ghosh
6. **Medical Management of Hyperglycemia in Type 1 Diabetes Mellitus in Girls** 36
   Rajeev Chawla, Shalini Jaggi, Aastha Chawla
7. **Insulin Injection Technique in Women** 44
   Sanjay Kalra, Sunil Gupta

SECTION 3: METABOLIC HEALTH

8. **Obesity and Type 2 Diabetes Mellitus** 47
   Anjali A Bhatt, AG Unnikrishnan
9. **Dyslipidemia and Hypertension** 57
   Anuj Maheshwari, Brij M Makkar
10. **Vitamin D** 63
    Gagan Priya, Rajat Gupta

SECTION 4: COMPLICATIONS

11. **Cardiovascular Disease** 71
    Mala Dharmalingam, Ganavi YP
12. **Diabetic Nephropathy** 77
    Vijay Viswanathan, Anitha Rani

13. **Diabetic Neuropathy** 81
Sweta Singla, Deepak Khandelwal

14. **Infections** 87
Jayanta K Panda, Madhusmita Patnaik

SECTION 5: ENDOCRINE HEALTH

15. **Polycystic Ovary Syndrome** 92
SR Aravind, Chitra Selvan

16. **Bone Health** 98
Ranabir Salam, Manash P Baruah

17. **Thyroid Health** 106
KVS Hari Kumar

18. **Eating Disorders** 115
Mudita Dhingra, Bharti Kalra

SECTION 6: GYNECOLOGIC HEALTH

19. **Contraception** 123
Beena Bansal, Parjeet Kaur

20. **Preconception Care** 129
Usha Sriram

21. **Breastfeeding and Diabetes** 138
Viveka P Jyotsna, Nishant Raizada

22. **Menopause and Diabetes Including Hormone Replacement Therapy** 143
Surya K Singh, Shweta Bhandari, Balram Gupta

23. **Malignancies** 151
Sudha Vidyasagar, Banshi Saboo, Anshul Singh

SECTION 7: PSYCHOSOCIAL HEALTH

24. **Sexual Health** 158
Rakesh K Sahay, P Venu Madhavi

25. **Anxiety and Depression** 167
Yatan PS Balhara, Arghya Pal, Sanjay Kalra

26. **Impact on Women: Having a Family Member with Diabetes** 174
Sanjay Agarwal, Shruti V Sheth

27. **Fasts in Women with Diabetes** 182
Sameer Aggarwal, Deep Dutta

Index *189*

1

CHAPTER

The Guidelines: Noesis and Hopes

Sarita Bajaj, Alankar Tiwari

INTRODUCTION

Diabetes has emerged as a global health problem and is rapidly gaining the status of a pandemic with over 415 million people affected across the globe. Women make up almost half of this figure in India as well as in the world. Figure 1 shows the prevalence of diabetes in South East Asia in different age groups in males and females. Recent data show that prediabetes is more prevalent in women and more women die of diabetes and its complications than men. Figure 2, highlights the disturbing mortality rates in women due to diabetes.

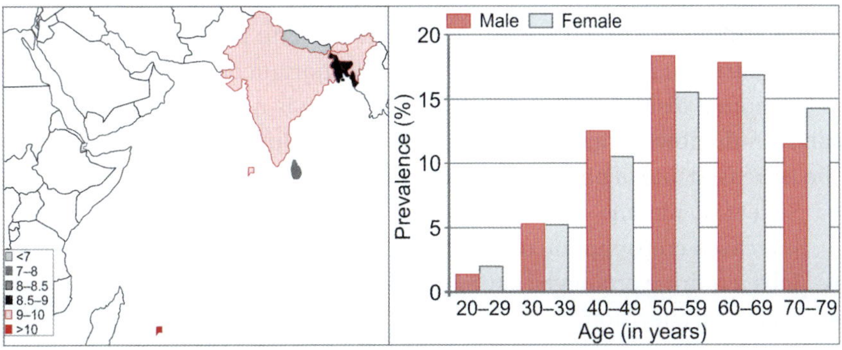

FIG. 1: Prevalence of diabetes in South East Asia (International Diabetes Federation Atlas 2015)

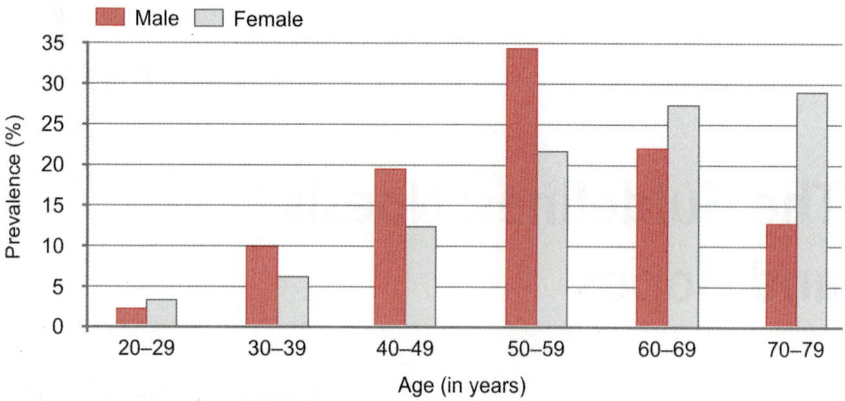

FIG. 2: Mortality due to diabetes, South East Asia region, 2015 (International Diabetes Federation Atlas)

INDIAN SCENARIO

India stands second in the world as far as the number of people living with diabetes is concerned and women make up almost half of this figure. This fact is strongly supported by the results of the Indian Council of Medical Research India Diabetes (ICMR INDIAB) study conducted all over the country to study the prevalence of diabetes in India. Figure 3 shows the age- and gender-specific prevalence of diabetes in the four representative regions of India.

Increased Prevalence of Diabetes in Women

This alarming rise in the prevalence of diabetes and prediabetes in women can be attributed to many factors; the most important being obesity. Obesity is no more a disease of the rich. In fact, obesity is now observed in higher ratios in the lower socioeconomic strata. The major factors contributing to the increased rate of obesity in women are:

- Sedentary lifestyle
- Increased consumption of fast foods and processed calorie dense foods
- Jobs requiring prolonged sitting
- Watching television
- Decreased manual labor due to availability of household gadgets
- Vehicular transportation
- Stress
- Polycystic ovary syndrome
- Use of oral contraceptive pills
- Gestational diabetes mellitus
- Genetic predisposition.

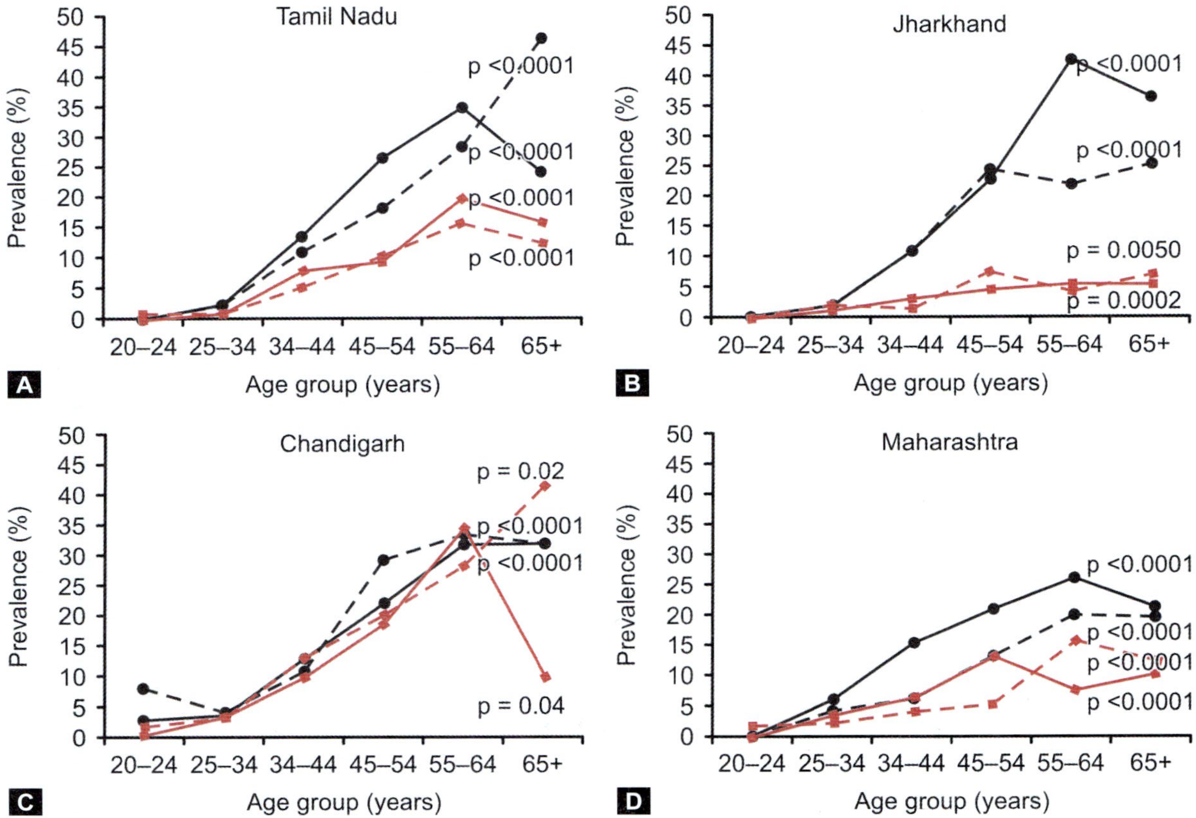

FIG. 3: Age- and gender-specific prevalence of diabetes in the four representative regions of India

In India, low literacy rates and increasing urbanization, coupled with traditions such as consanguineous marriages in certain communities, multiply the risk for diabetes. Cultural barriers additionally prevent the adoption of a healthy lifestyle.

How the Course of Diabetes Is Different in Women as Compared to Men

A woman's health poses unique challenges over her entire life span. Different phases of her life bring a number of physiological changes in the body, which affect the course of the disease in many ways. Puberty, pregnancy, lactation, and menopause are such chronological events in the life of a woman which add to the complexity of diabetes. Women are living longer and have added new roles to their traditional roles as homemakers and mothers. This has made women even more vulnerable to many lifestyle-related problems and to increased stress levels. All these factors make the course of diabetes in women somewhat more rugged as compared to men.

Cultural and Social Aspects Making Diabetes Care for Indian Women a Big Challenge

Women have been victims of gender bias at family and community levels and also at the level of healthcare delivery. The belief that girls are born to serve and boys to earn and rule, still prevails in most parts of the country. Gender discrimination begins from early childhood. In a limited income family, the boy is given better food and provided education. The girl child gets poor nourishment and is made to do household chores from a very young age. A woman in the family is placed at a low social status. She has no power to take decisions. This reflects on all aspects starting from the kitchen to raising children, and even healthcare. She is dependent on the male members of the family for healthcare interventions. For example, a woman may not receive needed healthcare because community norms prevent her from travelling alone to a clinic.

Women are often discriminated at even at the workplace. A woman with diabetes may be denied employment and may not be able to get a job of her choice. It is also a well-known fact that women earn lower incomes than men for the same job. A woman with diabetes may face difficulties in finding a good match for marriage. Lack of sufficient knowledge on diabetes can turn away a proposal. Factors such as future family life, pregnancy, ability to perform household chores, and the cost of treatment are all cause for concern when a woman has diabetes. On the other hand, it is easier for a male to find a spouse. At times, the disorder is not even disclosed. Illiteracy among Indian women is another big factor which contributes a lot to the negligence of personal health and nutrition, thus increasing the risk of developing obesity and diabetes many fold. An illiterate woman lacks the confidence to take decisions, especially regarding health problems and their treatment. Alternative therapies, wrong beliefs, and poor advice cause confusion, and she can be misled to seek wrong help. Besides, lack of knowledge on selecting a healthy diet and exercise accelerates the progress of obesity in women with diabetes.

Effect of Diabetes on Women's Health at Different Stages of Life

Childhood and Puberty

Type 1 diabetes mellitus (T1DM) accounts for 5–10% of diabetes prevalence and affects boys and girls equally. But in rural areas, and in many urban areas too, owing to gender bias, the girl child is neglected, and a girl child suffering with T1DM usually succumbs to it sooner or later due to acute complications like diabetic ketoacidosis (DKA), hypoglycemia, or poor nutritional support. They are neither provided proper pharmacological therapy nor nutritional management. Whereas girls in urban areas are exposed to junk and calorie-dense foods since early childhood in coalition with sedentary lifestyle which contribute to development of obesity. And this obesity makes them prone to diabetes in the near future. The most crucial and dramatic event in a girl's life is menarche and other related physiological changes. Hormonal changes during this period also affect the metabolic status. Body image issues, apprehension, and anxiety associated with menstrual cycles may contribute to increased risk of DKA and other complications related to T1DM.

Reproductive Years

Compared with the Western population, Indians develop diabetes at younger ages and due to this reason we are seeing more and more women in childbearing years with diabetes, including those women who go on to have diabetes during pregnancy (gestational diabetes). The challenges faced by Indian women with diabetes are unique and difficult. In addition to the medical complications of diabetes, with or without pregnancy, they have to face problems from the society and their families too. Diabetes during pregnancy has far reaching effects. Fetal and maternal complications can be very severe. The offspring of mothers with pregestational diabetes are at risk of congenital malformation. Women in South Asia lack preconception care, and adequate pre and post natal care. Women receiving care from trained birth attendants are 51% in India, 44% in Nepal, 27% in Bangladesh, 100% in Maldives, and 97% in Sri Lanka. A meta-analysis of 16 studies comparing preconception care versus nonpreconception care showed decrease in the rate of congenital abnormalities [2.1% vs. 6.5% RR 0.36, CI 00.22–0.59].

Women with diabetes during pregnancy have experienced unexplained fetal loss during late weeks of gestation. Moreover, the psychosocial aspects of diabetes during pregnancy cannot be ignored. It is very hard for a woman with diabetes belonging to a low socioeconomic strata to get proper nutrition and exercise during pregnancy. Many a times, a woman with diabetes may be pressurized to keep on getting pregnant in an effort to conceive a male child despite the difficulties of management of diabetes during pregnancy. Counseling and psychological support should be given to discourage such attempts. Sometimes, they may be coerced into sex identification and abortion of the female fetus. Proper family planning counseling and psychological support can help stop such practices.

Furthermore, the fact that diabetes is accompanied by increased vulnerability to develop tuberculosis in countries with high incidence must not be overlooked in women, since pregnancy can unmask this risk due to altered maternal immunity. Pregnancy is a known risk factor for the progression of retinopathy among women with T1DM. Also, women with diabetes lose their premenopausal protection from ischemic heart disease and have a risk that is comparable to that of diabetic or nondiabetic men. Women have worse survival and quality of life measures as well. They are also at greater risk for blindness due to diabetes than men.

In the reproductive years, diabetic nephropathy may be diagnosed somewhat earlier in women than men as nearly 25% of women with diabetic nephropathy are diagnosed during pregnancy. Women with preexisting diabetic nephropathy may have a marked increase in protein excretion because of the pregnancy-related rise in glomerular filtration from early pregnancy. This physiological phenomenon may increase the likelihood of earlier manifestation of diabetic nephropathy; although pregnancy does not seem to adversely affect the course of early diabetic renal disease. However, pregnancy accelerates the onset of end-stage renal disease in the presence of more severe impairment as manifested by hypertension and decreased renal function.

Postmenopausal and Old Age

In the current scenario, when life expectancy has increased substantially, women are living well into their seventies and eighties and spending a significant part of their life postmenopause. When women with diabetes undergo menopause, several physiological changes pose a big challenge for them:

- Menopause is associated with dramatic changes in lipids, body composition, weight, and increased risk for coronary artery disease. All these changes add to the metabolic and atherogenic changes that women with diabetes are already at risk for

- Menopausal women may develop vasomotor symptoms that may mimic hypoglycemic symptoms (sweating, dizziness, and hot flashes)
- In women with diabetes, already at risk for developing genitourinary infections, this risk increases manyfold postmenopause.

Elderly women with diabetes are at increased risk for bone loss and fractures. Prolonged fracture healing has also been reported. Diabetes increases the risk of dementia, vascular dementia, and cognitive decline. Social and economic issues will leave many older women living with diabetes alone and neglected.

Sexual Health in Women with Diabetes

Indian women often find their sexual health neglected due to social taboos and sexual dysfunction, posing a major complication in diabetes. An Indian study has reported poor knowledge regarding sexual function in women, but a strong need for sexual counseling, provided the healthcare professional initiates discussion. Most women report that doctors rarely discuss sexual health with them. One commonly missed condition is the vestibular syndrome (vulvodynia), which presents as dyspareunia. Sexual dysfunction adversely affects the marital life of women with diabetes.

Psychological Well-being of Women with Diabetes

Depression accompanies diabetes frequently and more so in the elderly and in women. Multiple factors play a role in the difficulties women face when diagnosed with diabetes. Depression and anxiety may pose hindrance in achieving good glycemic control and thus increasing chances of developing complications. These psychological issues also affect the family and social life of a woman adversely.

The Hopes Lie Ahead

Though there are many hurdles in the way of an Indian woman with diabetes in getting optimum care and treatment, many governmental and nongovernmental schemes are being implemented nowadays for upliftment and empowerment of girls and women which can be expected to go a long way toward raising the standards of healthcare for Indian women. One such scheme started recently by the Government of India is "Beti Bachao Beti Padhao" which aims to generate awareness and improve the efficiency of welfare services meant for girls. Other such schemes are "Janani Suraksha Yojana, Ujjawala, Women Helpline scheme, Indira Gandhi Matritva Sahyog Yojana," etc. Women are now being educated and informed about the importance of education and health. And, societal norms are now changing drastically and turning toward a phase of gender equality which will definitely enable Indian women to get the respect and rights that they are entitled to.

CONCLUSION

In addition to the problems faced by women with chronic noncommunicable diseases all over the world, women in India face certain unique challenges, on account of various socioeconomic, demographic, and cultural factors. They need to be encouraged to take charge of their diabetes and be empowered to make informed decisions, which will go a long way in better management of diabetes in this neglected population.

SUGGESTED READINGS

1. Bajaj S. ESI Manual of Clinical Endocrinology, 2nd edition. UK: JP Medical Ltd; 2015.
2. Bajaj S, Jawad F, Islam N, et al. South Asian women with diabetes: psychosocial challenges and management: Consensus statement. Indian J Endocrinol Metab. 2013;17:548-62.
3. International Diabetes Federation, Diabetes Atlas, 7th edition. 2015.
4. Kalra B, Balhara YS, Kalra S. Psychosocial aspects of diabetes in pregnancy. J Soc Health Diabetes. 2014;2:25-9.
5. Klein BE, Moss SE, Klein R. Effect of pregnancy on progression of diabetic nephropathy. Diabetes Care. 1990;13:34-40.
6. Misra A, Khurana I. Obesity and the metabolic syndrome in developing countries. J Clin Endocrinol Metab. 2008;93(11 Suppl 1):S9-30.
7. Mohan V, Kaur T, Anjana RM, et al. ICMR India Diabetes (INDIAB) Study Phase 1. 2016.
8. Ray JG, O'Brien TE, Chan WS. Preconception care and the risk of congenital anomalies in the offspring of women with diabetes mellitus: a meta-analysis. QJM. 2001;94:435-44.
9. Razee H, van der Ploeg HP, Blignault I, et al. Beliefs, barriers, social support, and environmental influences related to diabetes risk behaviours among women with a history of gestational diabetes. Health Promot J Austr. 2010;21:130-7.
10. WHO Country Profile. [online] Available from www.who.int/countrieswww.who.int/countries [Accessed July 2017].

2

CHAPTER

Women Hold Up Half the Sky and More

Bharti Kalra, Sanjay Kalra

INTRODUCTION

"Women hold up half the sky". Attributed to the Chinese leader, Mao Zedong (1893–1976), this phrase conveys much more than a mere demographic statistic, Chairman Mao has used this phrase as a wake-up call for women emancipation and gender equality. His choice of words conveyed that women shared equal rights and responsibilities with men. This philosophy led to significant changes in the role of women in Chinese society and economy. The phrase created interest throughout the world, and was used as a call to action in various media.

One platform which quoted this phrase was the book, "Half the Sky: Turning Oppression into Opportunity for Women Worldwide," by Nicholas D Kristof and Sheryl WuDunn. While these Pulitzer Prize winning authors and Zedong spoke in moral and socioeconomic terms, we use the phrase in the context of diabetes care.

WOMEN AND DIABETES

While diabetes is not exactly an "oppression," uncontrolled diabetes certainly is. Diabetes, however, is certainly an opportunity for women worldwide, to help themselves, others, and future generations. These facets of womanhood and diabetes are explored in the pages of this monograph, which seeks to investigate, interest, inform, interpret, and inspire. The aim of this information is to create a global movement, focusing attention on the special needs of women with diabetes, and highlighting the opportunities that they present for better care.

BIOMEDICAL ASPECTS

Diabetes impacts both boys and girls, men and women. From a biomedical perspective, however, it places a greater than fair burden on girls and women, on mothers and wives. Autoimmune disease occurs more frequently in the female sex, and this may lead to a higher prevalence of thyroid disorders in girls with type 1 diabetes mellitus. Puberty and menstruation add extra complexity to glycemic control in girls, who have to grapple with issues related to sexuality, contraception, pregnancy, as well as eating disorders.

PREGNANCY

The occurrence of pregnancy in preexisting diabetes, or new onset diabetes in pregnancy [gestational diabetes mellitus (GDM)] represents a major event in a woman's life. The fact that this occurrence is allowed to take place at all, however, is an equally major event in modern diabetology. While the pessimist is depressed by the ever-increasing prevalence, ever confusing screening strategies, and ever changing diagnostic criteria, the optimist finds cause for cheer.

Less than a century ago, pregnancy in a woman with diabetes was unthinkable. A diagnosis of pregnancy in diabetes was a death knell. By the year 1939, less than 1,000 cases of pregnancy in diabetes had been reported in world literature. The year, India alone is expected to have 4 million pregnancies complicated by GDM. With adequate medical and obstetric care, all these mothers should deliver healthy babies. If this is not cause for optimism, what is?

TRANSGENERATIONAL KARMA

Good control of diabetes, weight gain, and blood pressure during pregnancy contributes to better outcomes, not only in the expectant mother, but in the unborn offspring. This phenomenon, described as transgenerational karma, underscores the importance of women in diabetes care. Women not only support the present, they prepare the sky for our future generation as well.

PSYCHOSOCIAL ASPECTS

Diabetes in women impacts not only the person herself, but others as well. As a homemaker, the woman plays an important role in planning and fulfilling the nutritional needs of her family. She also influences the cooking practice and style of her relatives, friends, and colleagues. Coping with diabetes, in oneself, or in the family, allows one to function as a peer educator in lifestyle modification and diabetes prevention. This opportunity can be utilized as a public health intervention for primordial and primary prevention of diabetes. Women with a history of GDM, who have successfully transited to and maintained normal glucose tolerance are especially strong ambassadors of a healthy lifestyle.

WOMEN AS CARE PROVIDERS

Even when diabetes occurs in men or children, it does not spare the woman of the house. Changes in diet, physical activity, and lifestyle demand energy and commitment, which have to be shared by all members of the family. The brunt of this burden, however, sits upon the shoulder of the mother or wife. Women, therefore, do not just hold up half the sky in diabetes care; they hold up much more.

OPPORTUNITY

We do not consider this a burden. We view it as an opportunity to improve lives. Women are born with innate strength; this allows them to approach the "burden" of diabetes as a responsibility to be handled, apart from the multitasking that a wife and mother already deals with. With little bit of support from their healthcare professionals, women will be able to manage this more effective, and efficiently.

This book should be read on this positive note: Women with diabetes represent an opportunity to improve the quality of health, in themselves, their family, community and their offspring. We should make the most of this opportunity. For this, all stakeholders, including family, healthcare professional, society, and women themselves need to realize the importance of women. Women hold up half the sky, and more. They just need a bit of support.

SUGGESTED READINGS

1. Bajaj S, Jawad F, Islam N, Mahtab H, Bhattarai J, Shrestha D, et al. South Asian women with diabetes: psychosocial challenges and management: consensus statement. Indian J Endocrinol Metab. 2013;17(4):548-62.
2. Fraser A, Lawlor DA. Long-term health outcomes in offspring born to women with diabetes in pregnancy. Curr Diab Rep. 2014;14(5):1-8.
3. Hod M, Kapur A, Sacks DA, Hadar E, Agarwal M, Di Renzo GC, et al. The International Federation of Gynecology and Obstetrics (FIGO) initiative on gestational diabetes mellitus: a pragmatic guide for diagnosis, management, and care. Int J Gynecol Obstet. 2015;131(S3):S173-211.
4. Kalra B, Sridhar GR, Madhu K, Balhara YP, Sahay RK, Kalra S. Psychosocial management of diabetes in pregnancy. Indian J Endocrinol Metab. 2013;17(5):815-8.
5. Kalra S, Kalra B, Sharma A. Prevalence of type 1 diabetes mellitus in Karnal district, Haryana state, India. Diabetol Metab Syndr. 2010;2(1):14.
6. Nielsen KK, Kapur A, Damm P, De Courten M, Bygbjerg IC. From screening to postpartum follow-up–the determinants and barriers for gestational diabetes mellitus (GDM) services, a systematic review. BMC Pregnancy Childbirth. 2014;14(1):41.

3

CHAPTER

Overview of Women Specific Issues in Diabetes

Atul Dhingra, Kamlesh Ahuja

INTRODUCTION

Men and women experience diabetes mellitus differently in important aspects. Most of the current literature on diabetes mellitus has almost exclusively focused on men and the results of these have been extrapolated to women. Till 2006 no gender-specific guidelines for management of diabetes mellitus and its complications were available. This was probably because the recommendations were based almost completely on studies that either did not include women or were not powered by enough individuals of both sexes to assess the impact of sex-specific differences. Even when both men and women were included in studies, no attempt was made to assess the impact of sex-specific differences on the data. It has further been suggested that for optimal prevention and treatment of diabetes, these differences must be acknowledged. In past years, researchers have tried to specify the care of women with diabetes mellitus. This review is a comprehensive effort to integrate the information from these papers with a systematic survey of the literature about the sex-specific features of diabetes mellitus.

EPIDEMIOLOGY

Type 1 Diabetes Mellitus

The age of presentation of childhood onset type 1 diabetes mellitus (T1DM) has a bimodal distribution with one peak at 4–6 years and a second in early puberty (10–14 years). Clinic-based data from Haryana and Chennai have reported a prevalence of 1.02–2.60 per 10,000 children. Studies on Asian Indian children in the United Kingdom also have reported low prevalence of 4.8 per 10,000 in Leicester. Sex bias toward female population is characteristic of most autoimmune conditions. However, T1DM is different from other autoimmune conditions by virtue of its earlier age of onset and lack of female preponderance. In select population T1DM occurs more frequently in males. For example, older males of European origin are more likely to develop T1DM as compared to females of similar age group. However, studies from non-European population do show female bias.

Type 2 Diabetes Mellitus

Girls are 1.3–1.7 times likelier than boys to develop type 2 diabetes mellitus (T2DM) during adolescence. Although the reason for this increased risk in girls is not clear, it may be related to an increased risk of insulin resistance, as seen in adolescent girls with polycystic ovary syndrome (PCOS). However, this sex bias is reversed in adults. A study from rural Haryana showed higher prevalence of T2DM in males (15.8%) compared with females (11.1%), and the sex-wise difference in prevalence was statistically significant ($p < 0.001$). Most of the epidemiological data from west show a shift from female preponderance in studies published in 1930–1970 to similar prevalence in both men and women in recently published data.

PATHOPHYSIOLOGY

The natural history of T2DM generally begins with a constellation of findings related to insulin resistance. In women, the metabolic syndrome often includes PCOS, characterized by hyperandrogenism and anovulation. Girls have a higher (1.3–1.7 times) chance of developing T2DM during adolescence than boys. Furthermore, it has been hypothesized that mitochondrial defects are responsible for both depressed insulin secretion by β-cells and insulin resistance, particularly in skeletal muscle and the liver. Mitochondrial deoxyribonucleic acid is transmitted to offspring exclusively through the mother, which may help explain why diabetes is more often maternally inherited.

DIAGNOSIS

Diabetes is diagnosed when fasting plasma glucose is more than 126 mg/dL or 2-hour plasma glucose is more than 200 mg/dL. Because women are more likely than men to have isolated postprandial hyperglycemia rather than fasting hyperglycemia, relying solely on fasting blood glucose may underdiagnose the disease in women. Therefore, it has been recommended that women with significant risk factors for diabetes should have a 2-hour post glucose blood determination before the diagnosis is ruled out.

DIABETIC COMPLICATIONS

Neuropathy

Neuropathy is a common complication of diabetes associated with poor glycemic control. In a study by Lehtinen et al., the prevalence of symptomatic peripheral neuropathy in 132 patients with T2DM was 1.5%. Electromyographic abnormalities were more common in women with diabetes rather than control women, but no difference was found in men. Similarly, resting heart rate was higher in women with diabetes than in control women, but again, no difference was observed in men.

Nephropathy

It has been suggested that development of nephropathy in diabetic patients may be influenced by genetic factors, as supported by clustering of nephropathy in some families. Genetic factors may have a different impact in men and women. For example, the development of nephropathy in T2DM is associated in men only with the M235T polymorphism in the angiotensinogen gene (a threonine substituted for methionine at amino acid residue 235). However, a study from Joslin Diabetes Center at Harvard Medical School found that polymorphism did not affect the risk of diabetic nephropathy in women.

Urinary Tract Infections

Both symptomatic and asymptomatic bacteriuria are more common in women with diabetes as compared to men. In an Indian series, symptomatic infection was reported to be 14%, mostly postmenopausal women. In another study, asymptomatic bacteriuria was seen in 14% of diabetic women compared to diabetic men. Treatment for symptomatic infections is based on culture reports and a good glycemic control helps to eradicate the infection. Treatment is not indicated in patients with asymptomatic bacteriuria. Sodium glucose like traporters-2 inhibitors are also associated with increased risk of mild-to-moderate infections, more so in women. In background recurrent urinary tract infection (UTI), these agents should be avoided.

Diabetic Vulvodynia

Vulvodynia or vulval pain syndrome is usually described as "chronic burning," "knife-like pain," and "pain on contact" by patients. This is very similar to symptoms associated with symptoms of diabetic neuropathy. It has been hypothesized that diabetes mellitus may cause vulvodynia through many ways. Diabetes mellitus is associated with increased risk of vulval infections like candidiasis; it may also be a manifestation of painful sensory neuropathy or because of increased prevalence of other comorbid states like herpetic neuralgia in these patients. It has further been suggested that all patients with vulvodynia should be screened for diabetes mellitus and all women with diabetes must tactfully be questioned about vulvar pain. A detailed history and physical examination including cotton swab test or the Wartenberg's pinwheel to evaluate for hyperesthesia should be done. Diabetic vulvodynia is a diagnosis of exclusion and evaluation of vulvodynia must include an effort to exclude nondiabetic-related causes and must be followed by appropriate management. The mainstay of management is glycemic control, accompanied by pain modifying drugs as used in painful neuropathy.

DIABETES AND MENSTRUATION

Various studies have reported the interrelationships of the menstrual cycle and diabetes mellitus. Adolescents with T1DM have delayed menarche and a twofold increase in menstrual irregularities when compared with nondiabetic controls. In normally menstruating women with T1DM, both premenstrual hyperglycemia and menstrual hypoglycemia have been reported. Barata et al. evaluated the effect of the menstrual cycle on glucose control in six patients with T1DM using continuous glucose monitoring system. They reported that number of nocturnal hypoglycemic episodes was similar in the follicular and luteal phase but there was an increase in hyperglycemia (28.5% vs. 22.8%) in the luteal compared with the follicular phase. Goldner et al. who also used continuous glucose monitoring systems to evaluate glucose levels reported an increase in the frequency of hyperglycemia during the luteal phase. The authors hypothesized that glucose control seems to differ in the follicular and luteal phases, probably due to a hormonal effect or additionally to the presence of premenstrual symptoms or premenstrual syndrome, indicating that in women with T1DM the two phases of the menstrual cycle should be taken into consideration when planning insulin therapy.

DIABETES AND PRECONCEPTION

Preconception planning is the foundation for a successful outcome of pregnancy in women. Both American Diabetes Association and Endocrine Society recommend preconception glycosylated hemoglobin (HbA1c) of less than 6.5%. Preconception glucose targets of fasting capillary blood glucose concentration 80–110 mg/dL and 2-hour postprandial glucose concentration less than 155 mg/dL are reasonable to achieve an HbA1c level less than 6.5%. There is an increased risk of diabetic ketoacidosis (DKA) in women with pregnancy, primarily in T1DM but also in T2DM.

Women should be aware of this risk and the symptoms, management, and consequences of DKA. They should have ketone strips at home and be instructed to use them when blood glucose levels are more than 200 mg/dL.

DIABETES AND PREGNANCY

As per the 2013 International Diabetes Federation Diabetes Atlas, the estimated age-standardized prevalence (20–49 years) of hyperglycemia in pregnancy for India is 27.5% with 90% of women affected by gestational diabetes mellitus (GDM). A 2013 systematic review and meta-analysis of randomized trials for the United States Preventive Services Task Force found that appropriate management of GDM resulted in reductions in:

- Preeclampsia [relative risk (RR) 0.62, 95% CI 0.43–0.89; 72/1001 (7.2%) versus 119/1013 (11.7%)]
- Birth weight more than 4,000 g (RR 0.50, 95% CI 0.35–0.71)
- Shoulder dystocia (RR 0.42, 95% CI 0.23–0.77).

According to Endocrine Society, women with overt or gestational diabetes should strive to achieve a target preprandial blood glucose less than or equal to 95 mg/dL. Even a fasting level of less than 90 mg/dL is advised by some societies if that can be achieved without any undue hypoglycemic episodes. The target blood glucose levels 1 hour after the start of a meal should be less than or equal to 140 mg/dL and 2 hours after the start of a meal less than or equal to 120 mg/dL, when these targets can be safely achieved without undue hypoglycemia. The pregnant women with overt diabetes should aim to achieve an HbA1c less than or equal to 7% (ideally ≤6.5%).

DIABETES AND POSTPARTUM

All patients with GDM should be checked 24–72 hours postpartum for the presence of overt diabetes which was unrecognized prior to pregnancy. A fasting and postprandial plasma glucose of 126 mg/dL and more than 200 mg/dL is suggestive of overt diabetes. Treatment is warranted in these patients; the type of treatment (weight reduction, diet, exercise, and medication) should be decided on a case-by-case basis. Women who have fasting glucose levels below 126 mg/dL after delivery should have a 2-hour 75-g oral glucose tolerance test 6–12 weeks postpartum to test for diabetes or prediabetes. While any type of contraception is acceptable, as long as the usual medical contraindications to use are absent, intrauterine devices are preferable because of the minimal risk of unplanned pregnancy with these methods. Breastfeeding should be encouraged, as it benefits both mother and child. One prospective study reported breastfeeding decreased the incidence of diabetes 2 years after a diagnosis of GDM compared with not breastfeeding. Postpartum depression is more common among women with diabetes (pregestational or gestational) than in nondiabetic women. All diabetic patients should be screened for postpartum depression and patients with severe symptoms (e.g., suicidal or homicidal ideation with a specific plan and intent, or command auditory hallucinations) should be referred to an emergency department.

FEMALE SEXUAL DYSFUNCTION

Literature available on effect of diabetes on female sexuality is uncertain. Erol et al. evaluated sexual function in women with T2DM. They found that lack of libido was the most common symptom in diabetics and was observed in 77% of the women. Diminished clitoral sensation was observed in 62.5% of the women, 37.5% complained of vaginal dryness, and 41.6% had vaginal discomfort. Orgasmic dysfunction was found in 49% of the women. The incidence of all these related symptoms was significantly higher when compared to controls. The same was similar for women with T1DM. More women with diabetes than control subjects reported sexual dysfunction (27% vs. 15%; $p = 0.04$), but a significant difference was found only for decreased lubrication. No association was found between sexual dysfunction and age, body mass index, duration of diabetes, HbA1c, use of medication, menopausal status, or complications. Women with more complications, however, reported significantly more sexual dysfunctions, and the presence of complications altered treatment satisfaction.

DIABETES MANAGEMENT

There are no studies available that have reported gender specific effects of drugs available for diabetes management. Certain drugs like sodium-glucose co-transporter inhibitors are associated with increased incidence of UTI in women with diabetics. Insulin injections are commonly used in women with diabetes and injection through clothing is a common practice among women. This practice should be strongly discouraged as this leads to improper injection, increased risk of infection, and increased pain.

DIABETES AND MENOPAUSE

Available literature on effect of menopause or age at menopause on the presence of hyperglycemia is controversial. Most studies suggest that women after menopause have a higher probability of having hyperglycemia than men in the same age. A recent study from Japan reviewed data on 29,189 men, 6,308 premenopausal women and 4,570 postmenopausal women. The study reported that compared with premenopausal nondiabetic women, postmenopausal nondiabetic women, had a significantly elevated OR of 1.33 (1.20–1.48) for prediabetes; nondiabetic men had an OR of

1.93 (1.77-2.10) independently of age and demographic and metabolic factors. Even among women aged less than 50 years, postmenopausal status was significantly associated with an elevated OR [1.50 (1.18–1.91)] for dysglycemia (either diabetes or prediabetes). The reasons for this association are unclear. Furthermore, the author recommends that lifestyle modification in form of diet and exercise should be advised to menopausal women to mitigate this increased risk.

CONCLUSION

Diabetes is experienced differently by men and women. Unfortunately most of the available literature is based on extrapolated from studies done in men. Large studies targeting specifically these differences are needed for better control and care of diabetes in women. Gender specific guidelines based on these studies should be used for improvement in morbidity and mortality associated with diabetes.

SUGGESTED READINGS

1. Fitzgerald JT, Anderson RM, Davis WK. Gender differences in diabetes attitudes and adherence. Diabetes Educ. 1995;21(6):523-9.
2. Gale EA, Gillespie KM. Diabetes and gender. Diabetologia. 2001;44(1):3-15.
3. Heianza Y, Sone H. Response to comment on Heianza et al. Effect of postmenopausal status and age at menopause on type 2 diabetes and prediabetes in Japanese individuals: Toranomon Hospital Health Management Center Study 17 (TOPICS 17). Diabetes Care. 2013;36:4007-4014. Diabetes Care. 2014;37(7):e165-6.
4. Kalra B, Kalra S, Bajaj S. Vulvodynia: An unrecognized diabetic neuropathic syndrome. Indian J Endocrinol Metab. 2013;17(5):787-9.
5. Kalra S, Chandalia HB, Chawla M, Munshi N, Poojary A, Varaiya A, et al. Forum for Injection Technique 2.0 Addendum 1: Insulin use in indoor settings. Indian J Endocrinol Metab. 2016;20(6):863-5.
6. Kaveeshwar SA, Cornwall J. The current state of diabetes mellitus in India. Australas Med J. 2014;7(1):45-8.
7. Legato MJ, Gelzer A, Goland R, Ebner SA, Rajan S, Villagra V, et al. Gender-specific care of the patient with diabetes: review and recommendations. Gend Med. 2006;3(2):131-58.
8. Orchard TJ, Dorman JS, Maser RE, Becker DJ, Drash AL, Ellis D, et al. Prevalence of complications in IDDM by sex and duration. Pittsburgh Epidemiology of Diabetes Complications Study II. Diabetes. 1990;39(9):1116-24.

4
CHAPTER

Lifestyle Management

Ranjit M Anjana, Ranjit Unnikrishnan

INTRODUCTION

Women constitute half the population with diabetes in the world. Changes in lifestyle like sedentary habits, excess calorie intake, decreasing physical activity, and increasing weight are major factors leading to an increase in the incidence of type 2 diabetes mellitus (T2DM) in both males and females.

While the incidence of T2DM does not significantly differ between the sexes, women with diabetes face several challenges owing to gender discrimination and differential access to care. This is particularly so in developing countries such as India. Women with diabetes often struggle to maintain adequate control of their disease during the far-reaching physiological changes that occur during their lifespan. Epidemiological evidence also suggests a differential susceptibility to certain diabetes complications between genders.

Lifestyle modification (LSM) is an important means of preventing diabetes, as well as controlling it. This chapter will dwell on the specific issues faced by women with diabetes, with particular reference to patients residing in developing nations, such as India, in adopting healthier lifestyles that could prevent them from developing diabetes, and help them in better managing the disease once it sets in.

MAGNITUDE OF THE PROBLEM

The International Diabetes Federation estimates that, as of 2015, 415 million individuals have diabetes, out of which 50% are women. The gender differences in prevalence of diabetes have been shown to vary based on the stage of reproductive life, such that there are more males with diabetes before puberty, and more women with diabetes after menopause. However, in India, data from the Indian Council of Medical Research-INdia

DIABetes (ICMR-INDIAB) study, which is a national study on diabetes and prediabetes in India, suggests that until the age of 35 years, the risk for diabetes is similar among the genders (with the take off point being at the age of 25-35 years in both males and females). However, after the age of 35 years, the risk appears to be slightly higher in men compared to women.

The World Health Organization (WHO) lists diabetes as the eighth most common cause of mortality overall worldwide; among women, it is the fifth most frequent cause. Much of the excess mortality among women with diabetes stems from cardiovascular disease (CVD); it has been shown that these women lose the protection against CVD afforded by their gender and that their relative risk of developing CVD might even be higher than those of age-matched men.

LIFESTYLE ISSUES FACED BY A WOMAN WITH DIABETES DURING HER LIFESPAN

Childhood and Adolescence

Most prepubescent children with diabetes have type 1 diabetes mellitus (T1DM), an autoimmune disease with a unique male preponderance, and most nations, therefore, report larger numbers of boys than girls with diabetes. However, increasing levels of childhood obesity have led to the spread of the T2DM epidemic to children also, and the rate of this spread appears to be higher among girls. In India, childhood and adolescent onset T2DM is increasing and now beginning to be seen in the first decade of life especially among females in the urban areas. We have recently reported on a series of girls presenting with T2DM at 10 years of age or below. Whatever be the type of diabetes, puberty is a challenging phase for these girls. There is often deterioration in metabolic control consequent to the hormonal changes of menarche, and the situation is worsened by the development of eating disorders and teenage rebellion in some of these cases. There is also often a profound decrease in physical activity in adolescence among girls (see below), and an increase in calorie intake brought about by life stresses (school examinations and the like).

Reproductive Years

Diabetes affects around 1.3 million women of reproductive age worldwide. Most of these women have T2DM, but some are diagnosed for the first time during pregnancy—the entity termed gestational diabetes mellitus (GDM). Gestational diabetes mellitus is associated with various risks to both the mother and the baby. In addition, with the age of onset of T2DM steadily decreasing across the country, more and more women in India can be expected to enter pregnancy with varying degrees of glucose intolerance. While the pregnant woman in India can count on a considerable degree of family support, much of the well-meaning advice on nutrition and exercise offered by relatives and friends paradoxically makes control of diabetes more difficult, based as it is on myths and misconceptions rather than sound scientific evidence.

Middle and Later Years

Diabetes is a leading cause of mortality in older women. Because men with diabetes tend to die younger, there are usually greater numbers of older women than men with diabetes in most populations. Similar to menarche, the hormonal changes of menopause can also cause deterioration in diabetes control. Limitations in mobility imposed by osteoarthritis and osteoporosis may make adherence to lifestyle advice difficult at this age.

ISSUES IN MANAGEMENT

Apart from the management of diabetes, LSM helps in weight loss, control of lipid levels and blood pressure, mental wellbeing, and improvement in overall health. Unfortunately, women with diabetes, especially in developing countries, face several barriers which prevent them from fully obtaining the benefits of these interventions.

Healthy Eating

Women often face discrimination in their ability to partake of healthy diets. For instance, in many parts of southern Asia and Africa, men are considered the main breadwinners of the family and have the first access to superior (and more expensive) food. The women are considered as homemakers and have to make do with less than ideal food choices. For instance, in India, fresh fruits, vegetables, and protein constitute a much lower proportion of women's diets than that of men's. A much greater proportion of women's diet is made up of rice, as it is available at low expense through the public distribution system. High intake of refined cereals such as rice has been linked to increased risk of diabetes and makes the management of preexisting diabetes more difficult.

Physical Activity

Traditionally, women were occupied in nonmechanized domestic and agricultural chores and were able to keep themselves physically active without performing any specific form of "exercise". With the advent of household appliances and mechanization of agriculture, the scope for being physically active in the work domain has drastically come down, and this has not been compensated by a concomitant increase in recreational physical activity levels. It has been shown that only 10.7% of urban, and 2.9% of rural Indian women perform any form of recreational physical activity. Decline in physical activity levels is particularly profound after puberty in girls; results from studies such as the Obesity Reduction and Awareness and Screening of Noncommunicable Diseases through Group Education in children and adolescents (ORANGE) show physical activity levels to be equal among both boys and girls till puberty after which there is a rapid decline in girls.

Due to various social and safety issues, women in developing nations face several restrictions in performing requisite levels of physical activity. The barriers to achieving physical activity recommendations are myriad and include factors such as lack of time or a safe place to exercise, the fear of looking funny in exercise clothes, and (especially for women) loss of time spent with family.

A couple of examples from southern India show that it is possible to improve physical activity levels among women, although such improvements are often harder to achieve than in men. The Diabetes Community Lifestyle Improvement Program (D-CLIP) is a randomized controlled diabetes prevention trial in adults with prediabetes comparing standard of care to a culturally-tailored lifestyle education curriculum based on the United States Diabetes Prevention Program (DPP), plus stepwise addition of metformin when needed. Over the 3 years of follow-up, there was a 32% relative reduction in diabetes incidence in intervention participants compared to controls. In contrast to the DPP, the reduction in incidence was stronger among males compared to females. Men were also more likely than women to reach physical activity goals at each time point during the study. Women reported more barriers to joining the study initially, which might have influenced lifestyle changes. This reiterates the difficulties that women in India face in achieving exercise goals, even in the setting of a clinical trial.

The WINGS project (Women In India with GDM Strategy) aimed to address the rising prevalence of GDM in low resource settings. The project developed a context-adapted model approach to care (MOC) in low-resource settings to confront the widespread challenges in GDM screening and management, responding to the need to address some of the critical gaps in GDM care prevalent in low resource settings. The MOC was developed using best practice and established clinical guidelines, focusing on the importance of close follow-up and interaction between healthcare workers and patients. As part of the physical activity component of the MOC, all women with GDM were offered individualized one-on-one counseling about the importance and benefits of physical activity in pregnancy. Women were encouraged to meet the physical activity guidelines at every antenatal visit. Following implementation of the MOC, there was found to be a significant improvement in activity and decrease in sedentary behavior, with an increase in daily step count from 2,206 to 2,476/day. These changes were associated with improved control of glucose as well as better neonatal outcomes.

Issues in Access to Care

In many patriarchal societies of the developing world, women's health rarely gets the attention it deserves. This is especially so in the case of a chronic disease like diabetes, which involves lifelong medical care and frequent physician visits. In many parts of the world, women cannot venture out of the house without being accompanied by a male relative, even for a doctor's appointment. This often leads to missed appointments and poor compliance with the follow-up schedule. Also, social practices often prohibit male doctors from examining women patients; this leads to deficiencies in care when there is a scarcity of female physicians, as is the case in many parts of the developing world. The subordinate role assigned to women in these societies also means that they are denied the use of many of the newer (and more expensive) therapeutic options, when the household budget is limited.

PSYCHOSOCIAL ASPECTS

The traditional role of women in most societies is that of the caregiver. The alteration in this dynamic that occurs when a woman develops an illness can lead to considerable psychological stress, including feelings of guilt, worry about the future, and inability to cope. The situation is all the more complicated when the diagnosis of diabetes occurs during pregnancy. On occasion, these stresses may be of such magnitude as to push the woman into major depressive disease, with disastrous effects on glycemic control and self-care.

CONCLUSION

The woman with diabetes has to learn to cope with a chronic disease while juggling several roles—those of parent, professional, spouse, and caregiver. Among these competing priorities, self-care often loses out, with serious long-term effects especially in societies where the woman is traditionally conditioned to place family and society above self. Studies from India have shown that women tend to have lower awareness levels about diabetes, its complications and management compared to men. Women with diabetes need to be educated regarding the disease and the role of LSM in combating it. They need to be empowered to take major lifestyle decisions to attain their therapeutic goals, and provided with the necessary facilities to make these lifestyle changes.

SUGGESTED READINGS

1. Amutha A, Unnikrishnan R, Anjana RM, Mohan V. Prepubertal childhood onset type 2 diabetes mellitus: four case reports. J Assoc Physicians India. 2017;65:36-9.

2. Anjana RM, Pradeepa R, Das AK, Deepa M, Bhansali A, Joshi SR, et al. Physical activity and inactivity patterns in India - results from the ICMR-INDIAB study (Phase-1) [ICMR-INDIAB-5]. Int J Behav Nutr Phys Act. 2014;11:26.
3. Anjana RM, Pradeepa R, Deepa M, Datta M, Sudha V, Unnikrishnan R, et al. Prevalence of diabetes and prediabetes (impaired fasting glucose and/or impaired glucose tolerance) in urban and rural India: phase I results of the Indian Council of Medical Research-INdia DIABetes (ICMR-INDIAB) study. Diabetologia. 2011;54:3022-7.
4. Anjana RM, Ranjani H, Unnikrishnan R, Weber MB, Mohan V, Narayan KM. Exercise patterns and behaviour in Asian Indians: data from the baseline survey of the Diabetes Community Lifestyle Improvement Program (D-CLIP). Diabetes Res Clin Pract. 2015;107:77-84.
5. Anjana RM, Sudha V, Lakshmipriya N, , Anitha C, Unnikrishnan R, Bhavadharini B, et al. Physical activity patterns and gestational diabetes outcomes - The wings project. Diabetes Res Clin Pract. 2016;116:253-62.
6. Bajaj S, Jawad F, Islam N, Mahtab H, Bhattarai J, Shrestha D, et al. South Asian women with diabetes: Psychosocial challenges and management: Consensus statement. Indian J Endocrinol Metab. 2013;17:548-62.
7. Deepa M, Bhansali A, Anjana RM, Pradeepa R, Joshi SR, Joshi PP, et al. Knowledge and awareness of diabetes in urban and rural India: The Indian Council of Medical Research India Diabetes Study (Phase I): Indian Council of Medical Research India Diabetes 4. Indian J Endocrinol Metab. 2014;18:379-85.
8. Fagot-Campagna A, Pettitt DJ, Engelgau MM, Burrows NR, Geiss LS, Valdez R, et al. Type 2 diabetes among North American children and adolescents: an epidemiologic review and a public health perspective. J Pediatr. 2000;136:664-72.
9. Göbl CS, Brannath W, Bozkurt L, Handisurya A, Anderwald C, Luger A, et al. Sex-specific differences in glycemic control and cardiovascular risk factors in older patients with insulin-treated type 2 diabetes mellitus. Gend Med. 2010;7:593-9.
10. International Diabetes Federation. IDF Diabetes Atlas, 7th edition. Brussels, Belgium. International Diabetes Federation, 2015. [online] Available from: http://www.diabetesatlas.org. [Accessed March, 2017].
11. Kalra B, Sridhar GR, Madhu K, Balhara YP, Sahay RK, Kalra S. Psychosocial management of diabetes in pregnancy. Indian J Endocrinol Metab. 2013;17:815-8.
12. Kayal A, Mohan V, Malanda B, Anjana RM, Bhavadharini B, Mahalakshmi MM, et al. Women in India with Gestational Diabetes Mellitus Strategy (WINGS): Methodology and development of model of care for gestational diabetes mellitus (WINGS 4). Indian J Endocrinol Metab. 2016;20:707-15.
13. Mohan V, Radhika G, Vijayalakshmi P, Sudha V. Can the diabetes/cardiovascular disease epidemic in India be explained, at least in part, by excess refined grain (rice) intake? Indian J Med Res. 2010;131:369-72.
14. Ranjani H, Pradeepa R, Mehreen TS, Anjana RM, Anand K, Garg R, et al. Determinants, consequences and prevention of childhood overweight and obesity: An Indian context. Indian J Endocrinol Metab. 2014;18:17-25.
15. Weber MB, Ranjani H, Meyers GC, Mohan V, Narayan KM. A model of translational research for diabetes prevention in low and middle-income countries: The Diabetes Community Lifestyle Improvement Program (D-CLIP) trial. Prim Care Diabetes. 2012;6:3-9.
16. Weber MB, Ranjani H, Staimez LR, Anjana RM, Ali MK, Narayan KM, et al. The stepwise approach to diabetes prevention: Results from the D-CLIP randomized controlled trial. Diabetes Care. 2016;39:1760-7.
17. Wild S, Roglic G, Green A, Sicree R, King H. Global prevalence of diabetes: estimates for the year 2000 and projections for 2030. Diabetes Care. 2004;27:1047-53.
18. World Health Organization. (2017). Global Health Observatory. Leading causes of death in women. [online] Available from: http://www.who.int/gho/women_and_health/mortality/situation_trends_causes_death/en/ [Accessed March, 2017].

5

CHAPTER

Antidiabetic Drugs in Type 2 Diabetes Mellitus in Women

Ipsita Ghosh, Sarita Bajaj, Sujoy Ghosh

INTRODUCTION

Diabetes is defined as a group of metabolic disease which is characterized by hyperglycemia resulting from defects in insulin secretion, insulin action, or both. Chronicity of hyperglycemia may lead to damage, dysfunction, and failure of organs.

Diabetes in women is an upcoming subject and has lot of untouched areas of interest, which needs to be addressed. Diabetes is closely linked with women's health and also the reproductive life which includes pre-conceptional consulting, pregnancy, and menopause.

There are few important aspects of diabetes in women which has been established previously.

Cardiovascular morbidity and mortality is increased in diabetic women. This impact on diabetic women was studied in initial myocardial infarction (MI) survivors from Framingham Study and was found that with diabetes, women are at twice the risk of recurrent MI compared to men. Susceptibility to congestive cardiac failure was also found four times more common among women with diabetes (16 vs. 3.8%). Thus, it can be safely assumed that glycemic control is of utmost importance particularly in women. Postprandial blood glucose had a strong predictive power and is considered an independent risk factor of cardiovascular events in women with type 2 diabetes mellitus (T2DM).

In case of response to hypoglycemia, it was found that counterregulatory hormones were found to be higher in male. This was analyzed in three separate aged match randomized controlled trials (RCTs) using hypoglycemic insulin clamp:

1. Significant increase in epinephrine, norepinephrine, and growth hormone (GH) levels in males

2. Significant increase in epinephrine ($p < 0.05$) and GH ($p < 0.01$)
3. Significant increase in epinephrine ($p < 0.01$), GH ($p < 0.05$), norepinephrine ($p < 0.01$), and cortisol ($p < 0.01$).

The reason behind this dimorphism is possibly due to different glucose thresholds for counter counterregulatory release.

ORAL HYPOGLYCEMIC DRUGS USED DURING PRECONCEPTION

Fertility and Conception

Fertility is usually normal in women with type 1 diabetes mellitus (T1DM), but there may be delayed menarche in girls, especially if diabetic control is poor. Although the age at menopause in women with T1DM is normal, fertility declines with age when compared with the general population. Other potential causes are eating disorders and autoimmune premature ovarian failure which can be associated with T1DM. Polycystic ovarian syndrome (PCOS) is strongly related to obesity and regarded as a component of the metabolic syndrome. Women with T2DM are usually overweight and there is a strong association between glucose intolerance and polycystic disease. Subfertility due to polycystic disease responds to weight loss and metformin treatment. Other insulin sensitizers may also improve fertility but avoided due to possibility of adverse effects on the developing fetus.

Polycystic ovarian syndrome is one of the most common endocrinopathy in women of reproductive age, associated with adverse severe long-term health consequences due to diabetes, adiposities, and dyslipidemia. Oral antidiabetic drugs ameliorates hyperandrogenism and cycle irregularities with improvement in ovulation and pregnancy rates. Oral hypoglycemic agents, also improves insulin sensitivity, as insulin resistance (IR) is a key player in pathophysiology of PCOS.

A study involving 26 PCOS patients with 100% having irregular cycles and meeting ultrasound criteria, hirsutism in 90%, and high free testosterone in 85% showed that when put on 1.5 g of metformin for 2 months and comparing to baseline, waist-hip ratio (WHR) was significantly decreased ($p = 0.003$). There was also significant reduction in luteinizing hormone ($p = 0.0007$), total testosterone ($p = 0.004$), free testosterone ($p = 0.0001$), androstenedione ($p = 0.002$), dehydroepiandrosterone sulfate ($p = 0.006$), and the free androgen index ($p = 0.0005$), with increments in follicle-stimulating hormone ($p = 0.04$) and sex hormone-binding globulin ($p = 0.04$).

In another RCT conducted recently in a group of 84 females suffering from PCOS, randomly receiving one of the following for 3 months—metformin (1.5 gm/day), pioglitazone (30 mg/day), and combination of both metformin and pioglitazone—hormonal profile, fasting serum insulin, body weight, body mass index (BMI), menstrual history, and WHR before and after treatment were evaluated.

Metformin, pioglitazone, and combination therapy induced favorable changes in fasting serum insulin (39.7, 30.6, and 37.2%, respectively), homeostatic model assessment-IR index (44.5, 33.3, and 41%), after 3 months of treatment. Body weight, BMI, and WHR increased significantly after treatment with pioglitazone but the data were similar after administration of metformin or combination therapy (beneficial effect was mainly due to decrease in visceral fat). Total testosterone level decreased significantly only after treatment with metformin. After 3 months, in patients who received pioglitazone or combination therapy, menstrual cycles became regular in 71.4% and 73.9%, respectively. While menstrual improvement happened only in 36.4% of the patients treated with metformin. In this study, pregnancy rate on metformin was 10.7%, pioglitazone 25%, and 3.5% on combination therapy.

A meta-analysis evaluating acarbose treatment in PCOS demonstrated significant improvement in lipid profile, but an inconclusive effect on BMI.

Preconception Care

To prevent early pregnancy loss and congenital abnormalities in infants of diabetic mother, optimal preconceptional care should be started early.

Specifically, no contraceptive methods are contraindicated, so choice can be made by the provider.

Preconception care program includes:

- Counseling regarding risks and its prevention
- Selection of proper antihyperglycemic agents
- Establishing low risk glycemia without a risk of hypoglycemia.

According to National Institute for Health and Care Excellence (NICE) guidelines 2015, a woman with diabetes who is planning pregnancy should be advised to lose weight if BMI more than 27 kg/m^2 and should be put on folic acid 5 mg daily till first 12 weeks of gestation to decrease the incidence of neural tube defects in fetus.

Insulin therapy is the safest of all antihyperglycemic agents, but multiple injections and high cost reduces patient compliance. Oral hypoglycemic agents, especially metformin and glyburide, due to their ease in use, low cost, and safety profile has lead to its increase use in pregnancy.

Pregnancy

According to NICE guidelines, during pregnancy, routine follow up should be as given in table 1.

Table 1: National Institute for Health and Care Excellence guidelines 2015	
16 weeks	Retinal assessment at 16–20 weeks Self-monitoring or 75 g oral glucose tolerance test
20 weeks	Scan for structural abnormality in fetus—specially cardiac
28 weeks	Ultrasound monitoring fetal growth and amniotic fluid volume Retinal assessment
32 weeks	Ultrasound monitoring fetal growth and amniotic fluid volume
34 weeks	Nothing extra, just routine investigations
36 weeks	Ultrasound monitoring fetal growth and amniotic fluid volume
37 weeks	Offer induction of labor or LUCS in complicated patients
38 weeks	Offer induction of labor or LUCS in complicated patients
39 weeks	Advise women with uncomplicated gestational diabetes mellitus to give birth no later than 40 weeks

LUCS, lower uterine cesarian section.

Insulin Therapy in Pregnancy

Optimized pregnancy outcomes require excellent glycemic control. Limited by the dangers of hypoglycemia, current insulin therapies also cannot imitate the physiology required to maintain normal glycemic status. Evidence is literature regarding safety of current short-acting insulin (lispro and aspart) and long-acting/basal insulin is very little. Also there is limited information on the short-acting analogs lispro and aspart. Meta-analysis between lispro and regular insulin showed increase in large for gestational age (>90th percentile), but no difference in rates of small for gestational age with lispro group but has similar glycosylated hemoglobin (HbA1c) levels. Insulin aspart studied in another RCT along with regular insulin showed similar results. In both the studies, rate of hypoglycemia was less but not statistically significant in the analog group. Recommendation regarding use of insulin glulisine in pregnancy cannot be made as its use in pregnancy has not been reported. Regarding use of short-acting insulin and protaphane in pregnancy there is no safety information, but as its being used for long, it remains to be a standard comparator.

An RCT compared detemir with protaphane in diabetic women who were pregnant or in planning. Women receiving detemir at preconception had better fasting glucose levels along with lower HbA1c at 36 weeks. Women on detemir showing lower fasting blood sugar (FBS) did not have any increase in nocturnal hypoglycemia.

Studies on use of insulin glargine in pregnancy are retrospective and small, but shows no major adverse events as they do not cross the placenta. So glargine can be continued in pregnancy if required for glycemic control.

Absolute indications for insulin in pregnancy are mentioned in box 1.

BOX 1 Absolute indications for insulin in pregnancy

- Significant diabetes-related morbidity
  - High glycosylated hemoglobin
  - Ketonuria
- Significant medical morbidity
  - Associated renal dysfunction
  - Associated hepatic dysfunction
- Significant obstetric morbidity
  - Macrosomia
  - Intrauterine growth retardation
  - Hydramnios
  - Expected deterioration of glycemia control
  - Antenatal corticosteroid therapy

Oral Hypoglycemic Drugs Used in Pregnancy

Insulin has always been considered as gold standard for management of diabetes in pregnancy, which is mainly due to its effectiveness and safety which is unparalleled, and also there are no well-studied alternative. However, use of metformin and glyburide, has been supported by substantial amount of data. Insulin remains choice of therapy for higher levels of hyperglycemia, patients with significant obstetric morbidity (e.g., macrosomia, intrauterine growth restriction, hydramnios), expected to have deterioration of glycemia (antenatal corticosteroid therapy), and abnormal laboratory reports (e.g., ketonuria).

Current Place of Oral Antidiabetic Agents in Diabetes Management

The use of OHAs in pregnancies is not recommended by American Diabetes Association and Food and Drug Administration, whereas the NICE guidelines consider metformin and glyburide safe in pregnancy and lactation. The Endocrine Society suggests use of glyburide in gestational diabetes mellitus (GDM) only when glycemic control is not sufficient after 1 week medical nutrition therapy (MNT) trial. However, there are exceptions in cases with GDM less than 25 weeks and those with FBS more than 110 mg/dL—here insulin is preferred. Regarding use of metformin in pregnancy, it is used in unsatisfactory glycemic control on MNT and in those who refuses insulin and glyburide and are not in first trimester.

Metformin

A biguanide functions by:

- Increases insulin sensitivity
- Decrease in gluconeogenesis
- Enhanced peripheral glucose uptake
- Decrease in intestinal glucose absorption.

Three RCT regarding efficacy of metformin in pregnancy with comparison to insulin therapy shows nonsignificant but lower average fasting, postprandial levels, and HbA1c.

Safety

Maternal: Regarding safety profile women on metformin had significantly lower pregnancy-induced hypertension, weight gain, and rate of pre-eclampsia. Preterm delivery was significantly higher in metformin group and rate of cesarean sections had no significant difference.

Fetal: Placental transport—metformin crosses placenta freely.

Teratogenicity: Incidence of congenital anomalies in these studies were attributed to hyperglycemia during organogenesis and not to metformin.

Glyburide

Second generation oral sulfonylurea which increase release of insulin from the pancreatic ß-cells. Initial dose of glyburide is 2.5–5.0 mg OD/BD with a maximum dose that can be prescribed being 20 mg/day. Incidence of hypoglycemia being 1–5%.

Efficacy in pregnancy: Three RCTs comparing glyburide and insulin were reviewed and found that there was no differences in glycemic control between groups. A similar prospective study from India showed same results, whereas results from another RCT showed significant lowering of fasting and postprandial glucose in insulin group.

Safety

Maternal: Regarding safety profile rate of hypoglycemia in mothers receiving insulin, it was five times higher (20 vs. 4%) in one RCT study, but not in other two. However, all three RCTs showed rate of cesarean delivery were similar in both groups (23–52%).

Fetal Placental Transport: Placental transport of glyburide is significantly lower than chlorpropamide and tolbutamide. In an RCT study of glyburide versus insulin in GDM, glyburide was not detected in the cord blood of any infant.

Teratogenicity: In a study consisting of 147 women with glycemic control exposed to chlorpropamide/glyburide/glipizide, no association as found between congenital anomalies and use of oral antidiabetic agents. However, maternal HbA1c is an independent risk factor associated with congenital anomalies. A meta-analysis involving 10 studies on 471 exposed women to glyburide and metformin in first trimester showed no increase incidence of fetal abnormality or death compared with those unexposed but rate of neonatal hypoglycemia was significantly more with glyburide.

Fetal health outcomes: Among three RCT, neonatal hypoglycemia was significantly high among those receiving glyburide compared with insulin in one RCT, but not in the other two. Though birth weight was significantly higher, no significant difference was found in occurrence of large for gestational age babies in study groups.

During breastfeeding: Studies on breastfeeding is limited. Both glyburide and glipizide were not detected in breast milk and neonatal blood glucose was found to be normal with no incidence of hypoglycemia even when drug concentrations were at steady state.

Safety in offspring: No long-term study on outcomes in infants have been done.

Acarbose

Acarbose inhibits cleavage of disaccharides and oligosaccharides to monosaccharides. Hence, decrease in carbohydrate absorption in small intestine, and thus resulting in reduced postprandial hyperglycemia.

Absorption in maternal circulation is about 2%. No human studies on acarbose has been conducted though animal studies suggested no harmful effects, so use of acarbose is not currently recommended.

ORAL HYPOGLYCEMIC DRUGS USED IN LACTATION

Both first-generation sulfonylureas cross into breast milk. Tolbutamide less than 0.5% of the maternal weight adjusted dose. A 1 g dose of tolbutamide produced milk levels of 3–18 µg/mL in two patients. Chlorpropamide was found to be excreted in breast milk at approximately 10% of the maternal weight-adjusted dose. Motherisk study showed mothers on glyburide and glipizide failed to detect any of these drugs in breast milk though in a recent study, breast milk tested after 8 hours on glyburide was found to be less than 1.5%. Possibility of extensive binding of both of these drugs with plasma proteins may be the reason behind low transfer of these drugs.

Metformin

Three studies have been conducted in this aspect. One study revealed 0.28% maternal weight-adjusted dose was excreted in breast milk when mothers were put on 1.5 g of metformin. Second study conducted on mothers on 1 g of metformin was found to be less than 1%. A recent study was done on both breastfed and formula-fed infants born to mothers with PCOS on metformin (1.5–2.55 g) and results were found to be similar.

ORAL HYPOGLYCEMIC DRUGS USED IN MENOPAUSE

Increased Risk of Fractures

A Diabetes Outcome Progression Trial (ADOPT) study showed increased fracture rates in diabetic women on rosiglitazone. Subsequently, many trials confirmed this increased risk especially in elderly women on rosiglitazone and pioglitazone. Bilik et at. showed that postmenopausal women on thiazolidiones and men on both loop diuretics and thiazolidiones had an increased risk for fractures.

Thiazolidione exert its main metabolic actions through peroxisome proliferator-activated receptor-γ, regulates gene expression in adipogenesis, inflammatory responses, and glucose homeostasis. A series of experiments, in rodents, showed both rosiglitazone and pioglitazone decreases osteoblast activity and bone formation, with subsequent increase in bone marrow adiposity.

Mechanism of action:

- Number of signaling pathway at cellular level
- Decreasing insulin and amylin (anabolic to osteoblasts)
- Activation of peroxisome proliferator-activated receptor gamma leading to increased expression of adipocytokines has role in regulation of bone metabolism
- Rosiglitazone decreases circulating Insulin-like growth factor 1 level.

Results from ADOPT study showed diabetic patients on rosiglitazone has higher rates of fracture in women than in those patients on either metformin or glyburide. A pooled data on fracture incidence of patients on pioglitazone showed an increase rate of appendicular fractures in women on pioglitazone for maximum duration of 3.5 years, but an RCT study conducted in Japan showed no difference in fracture risk between these groups.[5]

Metformin, a potent stimulator of 5' AMP-activated protein kinase leads to activation in bone marrow progenitor cells and primary osteoblasts. Kanazawa et al. demonstrated metformin induced differentiation and mineralization.

Sulfonylureas are neutral to bone health. Monami et al. found no significant association of increased bone fractures with treatment with sulfonylureas, fractures risk tend to decrease. Kanazawa et al., found that postmenopausal women treated with sulfonylurea were inversely but significantly associated with fractures of vertebral.

Incretins enhances insulin secretion in response to ingested nutrients, plays an important role in bone homeostasis. Bunck et al, concluded that vildagliptin 100 ng for 1 year was not associated with changes in bone markers and calcium homeostasis when compared in drug naive.

Sodium-glucose cotransporter 2, Ljunggren et al. reported no significant changes in markers of bone resorption and formation.

Increased Risk of Infection

Sodium-glucose cotransporter 2: High glucose in the tissue promotes attachment and growth of candida, which is exaggerated in elderly women. There is also an increase in urinary tract infection with increase in osmotic diuresis due to its diuretic like effect in renal tubules.

CONCLUSION

Diabetes in women is an upcoming subject and is closely linked with women's health and reproductive life. Cardiovascular morbidity and mortality is increased in diabetic women, postprandial blood glucose being an independent risk. Response to hypoglycemia, counter-regulatory hormones were found to be higher in males compared to females. Fertility is usually normal in women with T1DM, but problems of delayed menarche, decline of fertility with age, eating disorders, and autoimmune premature ovarian failure is higher compared to general population. Polycystic ovarian syndrome a component of the metabolic syndrome has a strong association between glucose intolerance. Preconception care is of utmost importance, specially counseling, selection of proper treatment, and lower incidence of hypoglycemia must be taken care of. Pregnancy being a very sensitive issue, one should undergo regular follow-up with an optimized glycemic level should be our primary target. Metformin and glyburide can be safely administered along with insulin in pregnancy. Studies regarding glulisine and glargine are few, small and retrospective, and hence, not recommended. In lactation, second generation sulfonylureas like glipizide and glyburide can be used along with metformin. In postmenopausal women, increased risk of fracture with use of rosiglitazone and pioglitazone is a proven fact with metformin and incretins having a positive role to play in bone homeostasis. There is a risk of urinary tract infection in patients using sodium-glucose cotransporter-2 inhibitors.

SUGGESTED READINGS

1. Abbott RD, Donahue RP, Kannel WB, et al. The impact of diabetes on survival following myocardial infarction in men vs women. The Framingham Study. JAMA. 1988 Dec 16;260(23):3456-60.
2. Anjalakshi C, Balaji V, Balaji MS, et al. A prospective study comparing insulin and glibenclamide in gestational diabetes mellitus in Asian Indian women. Diabetes Res Clin Pract. 2007;76:474-5.
3. Briggs GG, Ambrose PJ, Nageotte MP, et al. Excretion of metformin into breast milk and the effect on nursing infants. Obstet Gynecol. 2005;105:1437-41.
4. Cavalot F, Petrelli A, Traversa M, et al. Postprandial blood glucose is a stronger predictor of cardiovascular events than fasting blood glucose in type 2 diabetes mellitus, particularly in women: Lessons from the San Luigi Gonzaga Diabetes Study. J Clin Endocrinol Metab. 2006;91(3):813-9.

5. Diamond MP, Jones T, Caprio S, et al. Gender influences counterregulatory hormone responses to hypoglycemia. Metabolism. 1993;42(21);1568-72.
6. Du Q, Wang YJ, Yang S, et al. A systematic review and meta-analysis of randomized controlled trials comparing pioglitazone versus metformin in the treatment of polycystic ovary syndrome. Curr Med Res Opin. 2012;28:723-30.
7. Elliott BD, Langer O, Schenker S, et al. Insignificant transfer of glyburide occurs across the human placenta. Am J Obstet Gynecol. 1991;165:807-12.
8. Feig DS, Briggs GG, Kraemer JM, et al. Transfer of glyburide and glipizide into breast milk. Diabetes Care. 2005;28:1851-5.
9. Gardiner SJ, Kirkpatrick CM, Begg EJ, et al. Transfer of metformin into human milk. Clin Pharmacol Ther. 2003;73:71-7.
10. Glatstein MM, Djokanovic N, Garcia-Bournissen F, et al. Use of hypoglycemic drugs during lactation. Can Fam Physician. 2009;55(4):371-3.
11. Glatstein MM, Djokanovic N, Garcia-Bournissen F, et al. Use of hypoglycemic drugs during lactation. Can Fam Physician. 2009;55:371-3.
12. Gui J, Liu Q, Feng L. Metformin vs insulin in the management of gestational diabetes: A meta-analysis. PLoS One. 2013;8:e64585.
13. Hale TW, Kristensen JH, Hackett LP, et al. Transfer of metformin into human milk. Diabetologia. 2002;45:1509-14.
14. Ho FL, Liew CF, Cunanan EC, et al. Oral hypoglycaemic agents for diabetes in pregnancy - an appraisal of the current evidence for oral anti-diabetic drug use in pregnancy. Ann Acad Med Singapore. 2007;36:672-8.
15. Holt RI, Lambert KD. The use of oral hypoglycaemic agents in pregnancy. Diabet Med. 2014;31:282-91.
16. Kalra B, Gupta Y, Singla R, et al. Use of oral anti-diabetic agents in pregnancy: A pragmatic approach. N Am J Med Sci. 2015;7(1):6-12.
17. Kalra B, Gupta Y. Pragmatic use of metformin in pregnancy based on biopsychosocial model of health. Indian J Endocrinol Metab. 2013;17:1133-5.
18. Lambert K, Holt R. The use of insulin analogues in pregnancy. Diabetes Obes Metab. 2013;15(10):888-900.
19. Langer O, Conway DL, Berkus MD, et al. A comparison of glyburide and insulin in women with gestational diabetes mellitus. N Engl J Med. 2000;343:1134-8.
20. Li XJ, Yu YX, Liu CQ, et al. Metformin versus thiazolidinediones for treatment of clinical, hormonal and metabolic characteristics of polycystic ovary syndrome: A meta-analysis. Clin Endocrinol (Oxf). 2011;74:332-9.
21. McElduff A. Insulin detemir in pregnancy: A small but significant step forward? Diabetes Care. 2012;35(10):1968-9.
22. Naderpoor N, Shorakae S, de Courten B, et al. Metformin and lifestyle modification in polycystic ovary syndrome: systematic review and meta-analysis. Hum Reprod Update. 2015;21(5):560-74.
23. Ogunyemi D, Jesse M, Davidson M. Comparison of glyburide versus insulin in management of gestational diabetes mellitus. Endocr Pract. 2007;13:427-8.
24. Pollex EK, Feig DS, Lubetsky A, et al. Insulin glargine safety in pregnancy: A transplacental transfer study. Diabetes Care. 2010;33(1):29-33.
25. Refuerzo JS. Oral hypoglycemic agents in pregnancy. Obstet Gynecol Clin North Am. 2011;38:227-34.
26. Rowan JA, Hague WM, Gao W, et al. Metformin versus insulin for the treatment of gestational diabetes. N Engl J Med. 2008;358:2003-15.
27. Russo GT, Giandalia A, Romeo EL, et al. Fracture risk in type 2 diabetes: Current perspectives and gender differences. Int J Endocrinol. 2016;2016:1615735.

28. Sehgal V, Bajwa SJ, Sehgal R, et al. Management of diabetes mellitus in the elderly with canagliflozine: A newer hypoglycemic drug in the horizon. J Pharmacol Pharmacother. 2014;5(4);227-31.
29. Sohrevardi SM, Nosouhi F, Hossein Khalilzade S, et al. Evaluating the effect of insulin sensitizers metformin and pioglitazone alone and in combination on women with polycystic ovary syndrome: An RCT. Int J Reprod Biomed (Yazd). 2016;14(12):743-54.
30. Tauchert S, Schröder AK, Ortmann O, et al. The use of oral antidiabetic drugs in the treatment of polycystic ovary syndrome. Zentralbl Gynakol. 2003;125(12):507-14.
31. Tempe A, Mayanglambam RD. Glyburide as treatment option for gestational diabetes mellitus. J Obstet Gynaecol Res. 2013;39:1147-52.
32. Valeria M, Maria CR, Elisabetta LR, et al. Gender differences in type 2 diabetes (Italy). Ital J Gender-Specific Med. 2016;2(2):60-8.
33. Vanky E, Zahlsen K, Spigset O, et al. Placental passage of metformin in women with polycystic ovary syndrome. Fertil Steril. 2005;83:1575-8.
34. Velazquez EM, Mendoza S, Hamer T, et al. Metformin therapy in polycystic ovary syndrome reduces hyperinsulinemia, insulin resistance, hyperandrogenemia, and systolic blood pressure, while facilitating normal menses and pregnancy. Metabolism. 1994;43(5):647-54.
35. Zhang YY, Hou LQ, Zhao TY. Effects of acarbose on polycystic ovary syndrome: a meta-analysis. Exp Clin Endocrinol Diabetes. 2014;122:373-8.

6

CHAPTER

Medical Management of Hyperglycemia in Type 1 Diabetes Mellitus in Girls

Rajeev Chawla, Shalini Jaggi, Aastha Chawla

INTRODUCTION

Diabetes mellitus is one of the commonest endocrine disorders affecting children. Type 1 diabetes mellitus (T1DM) tops the list of these chronic disorders, while other forms of diabetes such as early onset type 2 diabetes mellitus (T2DM), genetic defects of β-cell function, and maturity-onset diabetes of the young are increasingly being seen in this age group. With increasing prevalence of obesity, T2DM in young adults has become very common. Detection of autoimmune T1DM in adulthood [latent autoimmune diabetes in adults (LADA)] has also become common nowadays with improved genetic testing/genetic risk scoring.

Managing diabetes in children and adolescents can often be a tight-rope walk for the healthcare provider owing to certain unique aspects involved in the care of this delicate population cohort, more so in the young girls. Physical growth and sexual maturation cause marked variations in insulin sensitivity, more so at menarche and during the menstrual periods. Unique challenges to diabetes management in this age group include problems in self-care abilities, supervision in school or child care facilities, neurocognitive vulnerability to hypoglycemia and hyperglycemia, and potential comorbidity of diabetic ketoacidosis (DKA). The success of an optimal diabetes treatment plan depends on due integration of family dynamics and self-care capacity, developmental stages, and physiological differences due to sexual maturation. Due to a dearth of clinical research in this age group, the diabetes care recommendation in children and adolescents are essentially based on expert opinions and personal experiences rather than hard core clinical evidence or clinical trials.

This chapter addresses certain specific aspects impacting T1DM management in young girls.

The complex physical, developmental, and emotional needs of type 1 diabetic children necessitate management of this age group by a multidisciplinary team of specialists, sensitized and trained to deal with the pediatric age group and the various challenges typical to this cohort. Comprehensive care for them is an amalgamation of not only medical care but also psychosocial support, medical nutrition therapy, and structured guidance through diabetes self-management education (DSME) and support (DSMS). These should be provided not only at diagnosis but also on regular follow-ups, making comprehensive diabetes care a regular ongoing process.

Intensive diabetes education by an interdisciplinary pediatric diabetes team can arm them with the necessary skills and knowledge to manage their diabetes well. Hence, it is important to provide DSME and DSMS, medical nutrition therapy, and psychosocial support at diagnosis and regularly thereafter to these patients in a developmentally appropriate format that builds on prior knowledge by individuals well-versed with the educational, nutritional, behavioral, and emotional needs of the growing female child and her family.

GLYCEMIC CONTROL

The recommendation across all pediatric age groups is to achieve an glycosylated hemoglobin (HbA1c) goal of less than 7.5% (58 mmol/mol) as safely as possible with special consideration given to the risk of hypoglycemia in children aged less than 6 years because of their inability to recognize, articulate, and/or manage hypoglycemia. The link between recurrent hypoglycemia and delayed neurocognitive development in early childhood is well-established, necessitating the need to especially avoid hypoglycemia in this age group.

INSULIN THERAPY

Medical management of T1DM is centered on insulin therapy, with a variety of insulin regimes tailor-made to suit the individual, though not many have been specifically evaluated in children. Essential factors to be considered while choosing an ideal insulin regimen to meet the glycemic goals include the child's age, duration of diabetes, lifestyle and socioeconomic factors, as well as the preferences of not only the child and its family but also the treating physician.

Achieving glycemic targets with minimal or reduced hypoglycemia is currently possible with rapidly evolving scientific understanding and advancements using newer devices like ambulatory glucose profiling, sensor augmented insulin pumps with hypoglycemia suspend features, analog insulins, individualized goal setting, and basal bolus regimes as well as evolution of intensive structured self-management education protocols.[18,19] This has led to an increasing number of pediatric T1DM patients achieving their glycemic targets recommended by organizations such as the American Diabetes Association (ADA) and Canadian Diabetes Association (CDA), etc.

Further motivation for reducing glycemic targets has been provided by various studies documenting hyperglycemia related neurocognitive imaging differences. It is important to balance the long-term benefits of achieving a lower HbA1c against the risks of hypoglycemia and the developmental burdens of intensive regimen in children and youth.

GLUCOSE MONITORING

An essential arm of T1DM management is self-monitoring of blood glucose (SMBG) not only using point of care glucometers but also currently available glucose sensors that detect asymptomatic hypoglycemia as well as hyperglycemia, resulting in improved diabetes control. A randomized controlled trial demonstrated improved glycemic control in adults, though benefits in children and adolescents were not shown, probably owing to reduced use of sensors in this age group.

CHRONIC POOR METABOLIC CONTROL

Adolescence is commonly associated with worsening of glycemic control attributed to various factors such as adjustment and psychosocial issues of this age group, behavioral issues like intentional insulin omission, and physiological insulin resistance. Hence, a comprehensive multidisciplinary assessment for every child with chronic poor metabolic control (e.g., HbA1c >10.0%) is warranted to identify potential hurdles and etiologies such as depression and eating disorders. Modest reduction in HbA1c with reduced hospital admission rates have been demonstrated with multipronged interventions that target emotional, psychosocial, and coping issues.

DIABETES SELF-MANAGEMENT EDUCATION AND PSYCHOSOCIAL SUPPORT

It is essential to impart culturally sensitive, practically implementable, and developmentally appropriate individualized DSME and DSMS to young type 1 diabetics and their family/caregivers designed to suit their regional requirements at diagnosis and routinely thereafter.

Shared decision-making with youth and their family implementing recommended regimen and self-management behaviors is associated with improved diabetes self-efficacy, adherence, and metabolic outcomes. With variable cognitive abilities, "mature minor rule," is often adopted wherein children aged 12–13 years who appear to be "mature" have the right to consent or withhold consent to general medical treatment, except in cases where refusal would significantly hamper health and well-being.

An essential aspect of ongoing care is screening for psychosocial distress and mental health problems. The impact of diabetes on quality of life as well as the development of mental health problems related to diabetes distress include fear of hypoglycemia (and hyperglycemia), eating disorders, anxiety, altered behaviors, and depression. Children may be assessed for diabetes distress from ages of 7–8 years. Early detection of depression, anxiety, eating disorders, and learning disabilities facilitates effective treatment options and helps minimize adverse effects. An ongoing parental involvement in care throughout childhood with an adequate teamwork between the growing child/teen and parents/family further aids in better compliance and adherence. Healthy peer relationships and social adjustments at school aid in good school performance and academics. Suboptimal glycemic control may lead to poor school performance and increased absenteeism and disinterest in academics. Such children may need screening for depression and disordered eating behaviors with currently available validated screening tools. In children with eating disorders, it is also essential to look for weight issues and insulin omission behaviors.

Beginning at the onset of puberty or at diagnosis of diabetes, it is also very important to impart education about unplanned pregnancies and the increased risk of malformations secondary to poor metabolic control. Contraception should be discussed with all adolescent girls and women in the reproductive age group. Effective preconception counseling using developmentally appropriate educational tools helps adolescent girls to make well-informed decisions.

PSYCHOLOGICAL/PSYCHIATRIC RISKS

Children and adolescents girls with diabetes are increasingly predisposed to psychological problems and externalizing disorders as discussed earlier. An exponential increase in risk is seen during adolescence, especially with onset of menarche and during menstruation. Numerous studies have demonstrated psychological disorders associated with poor glycemic management and control leading to adverse medical outcomes. An increased insulin resistance at menarche and during periods is seen in young girls leading to worsening of glycemic control and increased insulin doses along with an increased propensity for psychological problems.

INSULIN RESISTANCE AT PUBERTY

Doubling of lean body mass over a period of 2–5 years at onset of puberty induces insulin resistance leading to increased glucose requirement and worsening of glucose control, which is further worsened by pubertal behavioral changes and psychosocial issues. A peaking of insulin concentrations (fasting and postprandial) is seen in mid to late puberty in both sexes. Compared to prepubertal and adult individuals, a reduction in insulin sensitivity by 30% has been demonstrated during midpuberty by hyperinsulinemic clamp studies. In T1DM, a similar exponential increase in insulin resistance has been seen in all stages of puberty. Hence, puberty is a time of worst insulin resistance at all stages showing an increased amplitude of pulses compared to normal subjects. The effect of growth hormone (GH) on insulin action at postreceptor level is well-documented. Hence, excessive surges in GH as occur in puberty, further contribute to marked worsening in insulin resistance at this stage. Hepatic GH receptor is partially insulin-dependent, so with decreased portal delivery of insulin seen in T1DM, the hepatic insulin-like growth factor (IGF-1) is reduced. A reduction in IGF-1 bioavailability also occurs secondary to reduced insulin-like growth factor binding protein (IGFBP)-3 and increased IGFBP-1 in association with waning insulin levels. Reduced IGF-1 activity increases GH secretion through this negative feedback mechanism, contributing to increased insulin resistance.

EATING DISORDERS

Ten percent of type 1 diabetic adolescent females meet the Diagnostic and Statistical Manual of Mental Disorders (4th edition) criteria for eating disorders vis-a-vis 4% of their age-matched nondiabetic peers. Furthermore, eating disorders have been linked to poor metabolic control and earlier onset and rapid progression of microvascular complications. These kids need early identification and individualized management strategies to optimize metabolic control and prevent microvascular complications along with addressing their behavioral issues.

PREVENTION AND INTERVENTION

Appropriate psychological evaluation and interventions in young female children/teens and their families have shown an improvement in their mental health, overall well-being and perceived quality of life, and alleviation of depressive symptoms. Evidence linking psychosocial interventions with better glycemic control, treatment adherence, and psychosocial functioning are fast emerging.

TRANSITION TO ADULT CARE

With time, these children grow transitioning from adolescence to finally adulthood warranting a need to changeover from a pediatric to adult diabetes healthcare team. This change of physician or diabetes healthcare team can have a major impact on disease management and metabolic control in these people. It has been shown that 25–65% of young adults do not have any medical follow-up during this transition phase and are more likely to experience hospitalization for DKA during this period. Hence, a well-organized and coordinated transition service may help address these issues and improve follow-up.

CONCLUSION

Childhood, adolescence, and emerging adulthood are periods of rapid and dynamic cognitive, developmental, and emotional changes. The young diabetic girl is faced with the challenges of not only maintaining good glycemic control in the background of her regular daily life, academics, extracurricular activities, socializing with her peers, and career choices but also the changing insulin needs secondary to physical growth spurts, sexual maturation, and varying psychological needs. Diabetes management during these phases of life places a substantial burden on the youth and their family, underlining the need for a multidisciplinary team offering a regular ongoing assessment of not only their physical well-being but also their psychosocial state and diabetes distress during routine diabetes visits. A well-balanced comprehensive diabetes management approach can help these young girls to transform into smart young women and walk towards a bright future as ambassadors of living a healthy life with diabetes!

SUGGESTED READINGS

1. Alam R, Sturt J, Lall R, et al. An updated meta-analysis to assess the effectiveness of psychological interventions delivered by psychological specialists and generalist clinicians on glycaemic control and on psychological status. Patient Educ Couns. 2009;75:25-36.
2. Amiel SA, Sherwin RS, Simonson DC, et al. Impaired insulin action in puberty. A contributing factor to poor glycemic control in adolescents with diabetes. N Engl J Med. 1986;315:215-9.
3. Barnea-Goraly N, Raman M, Mazaika P, et al.; DiabetesResearch in Children Network (DirecNet). Alterations in white matter structure in young children with type 1 diabetes. Diabetes Care. 2014;37:332-40.
4. Cameron FJ, de Beaufort C, Aanstoot HJ, et al.; Hvidoere International Study Group. Lessons from the Hvidoere International Study Group on childhood diabetes: be dogmatic about outcome and flexible in approach. Pediatr Diabetes. 2013;14:473-80.
5. Cameron FJ, Scratch SE, Nadebaum C, et al.; DKA Brain Injury Study Group. Neurological consequences of diabetic ketoacidosis at initial presentation of type 1 diabetes in a prospective cohort study of children. Diabetes Care. 2014;37:1554-62.
6. Campbell MS, Schatz DA, Chen V, et al.; T1D Exchange Clinic Network. A contrast between children and adolescents with excellent and poor control: the T1D Exchange clinic registry experience. Pediatr Diabetes. 2014;15:110-7.
7. Charron-Prochownik D, Sereika SM, Becker D, et al. Long-term effects of the booster enhanced READY-Girls preconception counseling program on intentions and behaviors for family planning in teens with diabetes. Diabetes Care 2013;36:3870-4.

8. Chida Y, Hamer M. An association of adverse psychosocial factors with diabetes mellitus: a meta-analytic review of longitudinal cohort studies. Diabetologia. 2008:51:2168-78.
9. Chowdhury S. Puberty and type 1 diabetes. Indian J Endocrinol Metab. 2015;19 (Suppl 1):S51-4.
10. Coleman DL, Rosoff PM. The legal authority of mature minors to consent to general medical treatment. Pediatrics. 2013;131:786-93.
11. Cooper MN, O'Connell SM, Davis EA, et al. A population-based study of risk factors for severe hypoglycaemia in a contemporary cohort of childhood-onset type 1 diabetes. Diabetologia. 2013;56:2164-70.
12. Corathers SD, Kichler J, Jones NH, et al. Improving depression screening for adolescents with type 1 diabetes. Pediatrics. 2013;132: e1395-402.
13. Delamater AM, Jacobson AM, Anderson B. Psychosocial therapies in diabetes: report of the Psychosocial Therapies Working Group. Diabetes Care. 2001;24:1286-92.
14. Doyle EA, Weinzimer SA, Steffen AT, et al. A randomized, prospective trial comparing the efficacy of continuous subcutaneous insulin infusion with multiple daily injections using insulin glargine. Diabetes Care. 2004;27:1554-8.
15. Ducat L, Philipson LH, Anderson BJ. The mental health comorbidities of diabetes. JAMA. 2014;312:691-2.
16. Harkness E, MacDonald W, Valderas J. Identifying psychosocial interventions that improve both physical and mental health in patients with diabetes. Diabetes Care. 2010;33:926-30.
17. Hassan K, Loar R, Anderson BJ, et al. The role of socioeconomic status, depression, quality of life, and glycemic control in type 1 diabetes mellitus. J Pediatr. 2006;149:526-31.
18. Hood KK, Beavers DP, Yi-Frazier J, et al. Psychosocial burden and glycemic control during the first 6 years of diabetes: results from the SEARCH for Diabetes in Youth study. J Adolesc Health. 2014;55:498-504.
19. Hood KK, Rohan JM, Peterson CM, et al. Interventions with adherence-promoting components in pediatric type 1 diabetes: meta-analysis of their impact on glycemic control. Diabetes Care. 2010;33(7):1658-64.
20. Kakleas K, Kandyla B, Karayianni C, et al. Psychosocial problems in adolescents with type 1 diabetes mellitus. Diabetes Metab. 2009;35:339-50.
21. Katz ML, Volkening LK, Butler DA, et al. Family-based psycho education and care ambassador intervention to improve glycemic control in youth with type 1 diabetes: a randomized trial. Pediatr Diabetes. 2014;15:142-50.
22. Korbel DC, Wiebe DJ, Berg CA, et al. Gender differences in adherence to type 1 diabetes management across adolescence: the medicating role of depression. Children's Healthcare. 2007;36:83-98.
23. Kuther TL. Medical decision-making and minors: issues of consent and assent. Adolescence. 2003;38:343-58.
24. Laffel LMB, Vangsness L, Connell A, et al. Impact of ambulatory, family-focused teamwork intervention on glycemic control in youth with type 1 diabetes. J Pediatr. 2003;142:409-16.
25. Lawrence JM, Standiford DA, Loots B. Prevalence and correlates of depressed mood among youth with diabetes: The SEARCH for Diabetes in Youth Study. Pediatrics. 2006;117:1348-58.
26. Lawrence JM, Yi-Frazier JP, Black MH, et al.; SEARCH for Diabetes in Youth Study Group. Demographic and clinical correlates of diabetesrelated quality of life among youth with type 1 diabetes. J Pediatr. 2012;161:201-7.
27. Maahs DM, Hermann JM, DuBose SN, et al.; DPV Initiative; T1D Exchange Clinic Network. Contrasting the clinical care and outcomes of 2,622 children with type 1 diabetes less than 6 years of age in the United States T1D Exchange and German/Austrian DPV registries. Diabetologia. 2014;57:1578-85.

28. Markowitz JT, Butler DA, Volkening LK, et al. Brief screening tool for disordered eating in diabetes: internal consistency and external validity in a contemporary sample of pediatric patients with type 1 diabetes. Diabetes Care. 2010;33:495-500.
29. Markowitz JT, Garvey KC, Laffel LMB. Developmental changes in the roles of patients and families in type 1 diabetes management. Curr Diabetes Rev. 2015;11:231-8.
30. McCarthy AM, Lindgren S, Mengeling MA, et al. Factors associated with academic achievement in children with type 1 diabetes. Diabetes Care. 2003;26:112-7.
31. Nakhla M, Daneman D, To T, et al. Transition to adult care for youths with diabetes mellitus: findings from a Universal Health Care System. Pediatrics. 2009;124:e1134-41.
32. Nimri R, Weintrob N, Benzaquen H, et al. Insulin pump therapy in youth with type 1 diabetes: a retrospective paired study. Pediatrics. 2006;117:2126-31.
33. Nordly S, Mortensen HB, Andreasen AH. Factors associated with glycaemic outcome of childhood diabetes care in Denmark. Diabet Med. 2005;22:1566-73.
34. Oram RA, Patel K, Hill A, et al. A type 1 diabetes genetic risk score can aid discrimination between type 1 and type 2 diabetes in young adults. Diabetes Care. 2016;39:337-44.
35. Pacaud D, Yale JF, Stephure D. Problems in transition from pediatric care to adult care for individuals with diabetes. Can J Diabetes. 2005;29:13-8.
36. Rosenbauer J, Dost A, Karges B, et al.; DPV Initiative and the German BMBF Competence Network Diabetes Mellitus. Improved metabolic control in children and adolescents with type 1 diabetes: a trend analysis using prospective multicenter data from Germany and Austria. Diabetes Care. 2012;35:80-6.
37. Swift PGF, Skinner TC, de Beaufort CE, et al.; Hvidoere Study Group on Childhood Diabetes. Target setting in intensive insulin management is associated with metabolic control: the Hvidoere Childhood Diabetes Study Group Centre Differences Study 2005. Pediatr Diabetes. 2010;11:271-8.
38. Tamborlane WV, Beck RW, Bode BW. Juvenile Diabetes Research Foundation Continuous Glucose Monitoring Study Group Continuous glucose monitoring and intensive treatment of type 1 diabetes. N Engl J Med. 2008;359:1464-76.
39. van Walleghem N, Macdonald CA, Dean HJ. Evaluation of a systems navigator model for transition from pediatric to adult care for young adults with type 1 diabetes. Diabetes Care. 2008;31:1529-30.
40. Wherrett D, Huot C, Mitchell B, et al. Type 1 Diabetes in Children and Adolescents Canadian Diabetes Association Clinical Practice Guidelines Expert Committee 2016.
41. Winkley K, Ismail K, Landau S. Psychological interventions to improve glycaemic control in patients with type 1 diabetes: systematic review and meta-analysis of randomised controlled trials. BMJ. 2006;333:65.
42. Wisting L, Frøisland DH, Skrivarhaug T, et al. Disturbed eating behavior and omission of insulin in adolescents receiving intensified insulin treatment: a nationwide population-based study. Diabetes Care. 2013;36:3382-7.
43. Young-Hyman D, de Groot M, Hill-Briggs F, et al. Psychosocial care for people with diabetes: a position statement of the American Diabetes Association. Diabetes Care. 2016;39:2126-40.
44. Young-Hyman DL, Davis CL. Disordered eating behavior in individuals with diabetes. importance of context, evaluation, and classification. Diabetes Care. 2010;33:683-9.

7

CHAPTER

Insulin Injection Technique in Women

Sanjay Kalra, Sunil Gupta

INTRODUCTION

Insulin injection technique is similar in women and men. However, subtle physiological, biomedical, and psychosocial differences are discussed in this chapter.

These include:

- Physiological difference in subcutaneous tissue thickness
- Preconception counseling in type 1 and type 2 diabetes mellitus
- Insulin injection sites during pregnancy
- Social barriers to choice of injection site
- Injection through clothing.

LOCAL SITE REACTIONS

The Insulin Technique Questionnaire (ITQ) survey included 1,011 participants from India, of whom 43.8% were female, and 0.5% had gestational diabetes mellitus (GDM). No sex-related differences in insulin technique or complications were noted in this study. In fact, women are reported to have thicker subcutaneous tissue than men, over most sites and body mass index ranges. This may reduce the risk of inadvertent intramuscular injection in women. There is no reported gender difference in the prevalence of local site reactions with insulin injection. However, women may find some adverse events, such as bruising, ecchymosis, and hyperpigmentation, socially troublesome.

PRECONCEPTION

Women with preexisting type 1 or type 2 diabetes mellitus need to undergo preconception counseling, which may include initiation or intensification of insulin therapy. This opportunity must be utilized to revise insulin technique and inspect palpable injection sites for local site reactions. Gestational diabetes mellitus complicates every sixth pregnancy. Of all women with GDM, about 10% need insulin. The screening and diagnosis of GDM should be accompanied by counseling regarding the possible need for insulin therapy. If insulin is initiated, adequate attention should be paid to allay diabetes distress, including concern regarding insulin use.

INJECTION SITES DURING PREGNANCY

During pregnancy, some women may display apprehension in injecting over the abdomen. They must be reassured that subcutaneous tissue does not thin out during gestation. However, skin near the umbilicus, taut skin, stretch marks, and surgical scar marks must be avoided. The Forum for Injection Technique 2.0 India guidelines suggest the following sites for insulin injection:

- First trimester: Usual sites
- Second trimester: Lateral parts of the abdomen
- Third trimester: Lateral parts of the abdomen, with raised skin fold; upper arm; thigh.

SOCIAL BARRIERS

Many women, especially in India, face social barriers to insulin injection in public places. For women who are unable to expose the thigh or abdomen, the upper arm is an acceptable injection site.

However, effects must be made to offer privacy for insulin injections in all public places. Women may find it convenient to wear loose fitting clothing which can be folded back to expose appropriate injection sites. Injection through clothing must be firmly discouraged.

In busy clinics, it may be difficult for the diabetes caregiver to provide privacy in order to palpate the abdomen and detect lipohypertrophy. Such facilities should be created wherever possible. A socially acceptable alternative is to encourage women to take photographs of their insulin injection sites (self-IE = self-insulin site examination), this can serve as a screening tool for detection of local sites reactions.

CONCLUSION

Girls and women may face gender-specific challenges with regard to insulin technique. Awareness of these issues, coupled with empathic and sensitive addressal, can help facilitate optimal insulin delivery in such persons.

SUGGESTED READINGS

1. Bajaj S, Jawad F, Islam N, et al. South Asian women with diabetes: psychosocial challenges and management: consensus statement. Indian J Endocrinol Metab. 2013;17(4):54862.
2. Billionnet C, Mitanchez D, Weill A, et al. Gestational diabetes and adverse perinatal outcomes from 7,16,152 births in France in 2012. Diabetologia. 2017;60(4):636-44.
2. Frid AH, Kreugel G, Grassi G, et al. New insulin delivery recommendations. Mayo Clin Proc. 2016;91(9):1231-55.
3. Jain SM, Pandey K, Lahoti A, et al. Evaluation of skin and subcutaneous tissue thickness at insulin injection sites in Indian, insulin naïve, type-2 diabetic adult population. Indian J Endocrinol Metab. 2013;17(5):864-70.
4. Kalra B, Gupta Y, Kalra S. Pre-conception management of diabetes. J Pak Med Assoc. 2015;65(11):1242-3.
5. Kalra S, Mithal A, Sahay R, et al. Indian injection technique study: injecting complications, education, and the health care professional. Diabetes Ther. 2017:1-4.
6. Kalra S, Mithal A, Sahay R, et al. Indian injection technique study: population characteristics and injection practices. Diabetes Ther. 2017:1-21.
7. Tandon N, Kalra S, Balhara YS, et al. Forum for injection technique (FIT), India: The Indian recommendations 2.0, for best practice in Insulin Injection Technique, 2015. Indian J Endocrinol Metab. 2015;19:317-31.

8
CHAPTER

Obesity and Type 2 Diabetes Mellitus

Anjali A Bhatt, AG Unnikrishnan

INTRODUCTION

While both women and men share some similar health challenges, some differences make women's health deserve particular attention. Biologically, women have a survival advantage in that they live longer than men but in developing countries these advantages are often overridden by gender-based discrimination, making female life expectancy at birth lower than or equal to that of males. In these settings even the longer lives are not often healthy lives. Certain biological events (e.g., pregnancy, childbirth, and breastfeeding) are experienced only by women in their lifetime and may negatively impact their health if proper care is not provided. Women are not only physiologically different than men but there are also social, ethnic, and cultural differences making women more vulnerable to many diseases—especially in India. One of the most concerning disease reaching epidemic proportions globally in both men and women is obesity and the consequent type 2 diabetes mellitus (T2DM). According to global data, women are clearly at a higher risk of obesity and the consequent T2DM. Obese women are at risk of developing diabetes which is 12 times higher than the risk of a normal weight woman. Ironically in India, prevalence of both obesity and nutritional deficiencies is more common in women compared to men.

EPIDEMIOLOGICAL PERSPECTIVE

Epidemiological studies have given a grave picture of epidemic proportions of T2DM worldwide and the prevalence is expected to increase exponentially in the coming years. The global prevalence of diabetes is expected to increase by more than 100% with a huge variation based on ethnicity, geography, and gender. By 2050, rate of this increase is expected

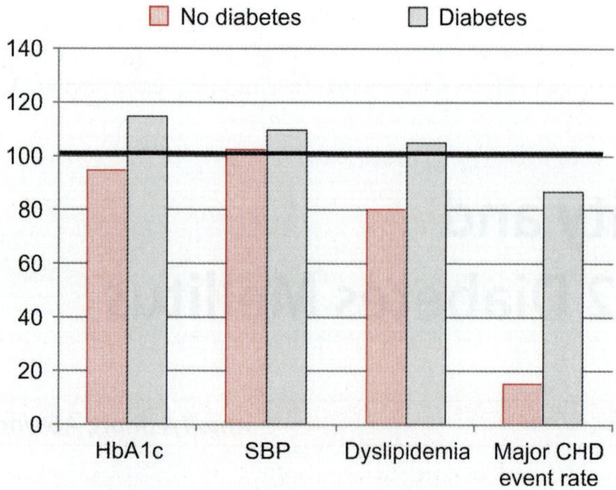

HbA1c, glycosylated hemoglobin; SBP, systolic blood pressure.

FIG. 1: Level of risk factors and coronary heart disease event rate in women compared to men (men = 100%)

to be more in women (220%) than in men (174%), particularly for Indian women. A recent systematic review on Asian Indian reported that the prevalence of obesity in women in higher than in men. Interestingly, the diabetes-related risk factors which are found to be at a lower rate in nondiabetic women are increased exponentially in women with diabetes, compared to men as shown in figure 1.

What, then are the factors responsible for these disparities? The underlying pathophysiology of diabetes is diverse and is affected by genetics, body composition, basal metabolic rate, and lifestyle (diet, physical activity, and stress). These factors in addition to factors like cultural, socioeconomic, and healthcare access also influence the health outcomes and complications from diabetes. A number of factors differentiate Indian women and predispose them to obesity namely, sedentary behavior, unhealthy diets, sequential and additive postpartum weight gain (mainly secondary to wrong beliefs regarding diet during pregnancy and lactation), and further decrease in physical activity during this period. An average increase in body mass index (BMI) by 2 units in a follow-up period of 4 years is seen in women aged 15–49 years. Healthcare access is also more difficult to women compared to men in India—especially the preventive health care.

As such it is not uncommon in India to find neglect of woman's health (mainly diet and devoting time for physical activity) by herself, by the family, as well as by the society. In fact studies on Western population too have shown that men are likely to eat more fruits, more fibers, and are likely to be more active compared to women. These results are definitely not generalizable but suggest the behavioral differences between the genders. India is in the transition towards social and technological development.

A change in diet and physical activity with a generations old background of maternal malnutrition poses a double burden in making Indian youth more prone for abnormalities in glucose metabolism. An example of this is an improved social and economic status but four times higher prevalence of overweight and obesity in women with 12 or more years of schooling education and 10 times higher prevalence of obesity in women with "highest wealth index" compared to "lowest health index" in spite of better access to healthy food. The proportion of overweight or obesity also varies from different states in the country making a generalized nutritional strategy less useful.

PATHOPHYSIOLOGICAL PERSPECTIVE

Estrogens are responsible for regulation of body composition, energy balance, and insulin sensitivity in both women and men. They not only regulate the satiety through central as well as local hormones but also increase the hepatic insulin sensitivity and pancreatic beta cell function. Physiologically women are thought to be protected from the metabolic abnormalities due to distribution of more fat in subcutaneous depots compared to visceral depots regulated by estrogen—this protections is lost after cessation of endogenous estrogen production following menopause. However, results of trials studying association of endogenous sex hormones (mainly testosterone and the estrogen estradiol) with diabetes and metabolic syndrome in women are equivocal. And, in reality, prevalence of both diabetes as well as obesity is higher even in premenopausal women compared to men. This observation in addition to the biochemical proofs from large population-based trials suggest that the metabolic abnormality secondary to insulin resistance associated with adiposity are overwhelmingly more powerful than the effects of androgens. It is also postulated that the relationship between sex steroids and glucose metabolism may be different in obese women compared to the lean ones.

PRACTICAL PERSPECTIVE

As mentioned earlier, women undergo a biological turmoil during their lifetime which is further intensified by cultural beliefs related to the stages of women's life in India. No wonder, diabetes is affecting almost every step of a woman's life including adolescence (and puberty), conception, childbearing, childbirth, breastfeeding, and finally menopausal as well as the postmenopausal life. Figure 2 depicts various stages of a woman's life which are affected by obesity and metabolic abnormalities especially T2DM.

Further in this chapter, case-based scenarios related to obesity and T2DM in a women's lifetime are discussed which are representation of common practical challenges faced by the treating doctors.

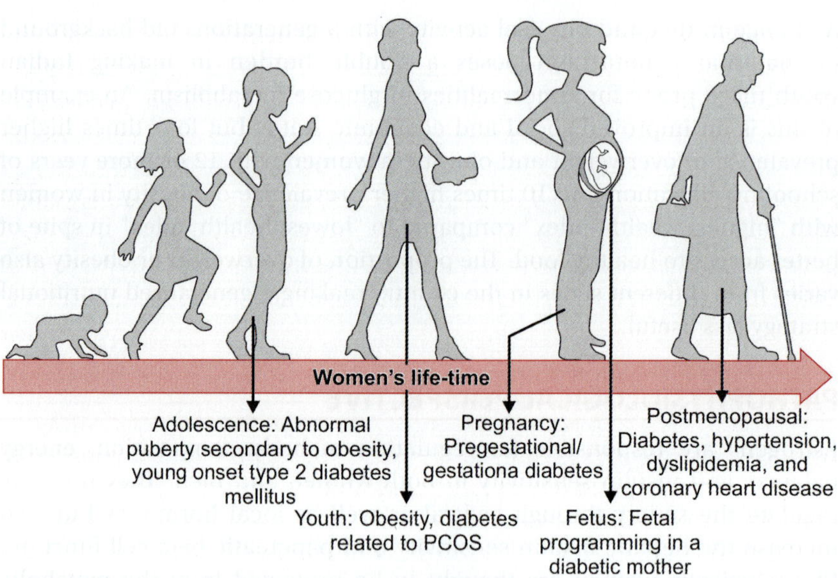

PCOS, polycystic ovary syndrome.

FIG. 2: Various stages of a woman's lifetime

Scenario 1

A 14-year-old obese girl, attained menarche at 10 years was brought by her parents for complaints of menstrual irregularities. On examination she was obese, had hirsutism, acanthosis nigricans, and on investigations was found to have diabetes mellitus.

Type 2 diabetes mellitus is not as rare in youth as was thought earlier. A recent population-based study found an overall prevalence of dysglycemia among children and adolescents in urban South India to be 3.7% and as high as 12.7% in girls with abdominal obesity. Type 2 diabetes mellitus in children is often associated with other features of insulin resistance (hallmark of T2DM) like visceral obesity, acanthosis nigricans, hyperlipidemia, fatty liver, ovarian hyperandrogenism in girls, and a strong family history of T2DM. Type 2 diabetes mellitus in children manifests itself most often during the second decade of life (~13.5 years); which coincides with the physiological peak in insulin resistance during puberty. Two points to note here are: (i) puberty may unmask diabetes in previously compensated adolescents to become overt and (ii) once the pubertal phase is over, these children may have a better control of metabolic parameters. Girls with insulin resistance may present with one or more features of metabolic (diabetes, hyperlipidemia, hypertension) and/or hormonal (early puberty, menstrual irregularity, and hirsutism) abnormalities. Reproductive abnormalities may be perceived as immediately distressing and are likely to be addressed more readily than the metabolic abnormalities which pose a long-term but definite cardiovascular risk. The evaluation should focus on testing blood pressure, blood glucose, lipid levels, and urine albumin in addition to the reproductive evaluation. A gynecologist is usually the first point of contact, hence would be important in such an evaluation. A strong advice for weight loss with lifestyle modifications is recommended. Metformin may be added for impaired glucose levels or diabetes and may also help to restore menstrual cyclicity and ovulation. Antihypertensive and lipid lowering medications may be added if lifestyle modifications are not sufficient.

Scenario 2

A 28-year-old lady who is known to have impaired fasting glucose and polycystic ovarian syndrome (PCOS), presented for inability to conceive even after 2 years of marriage.

The next challenge after "teen age" in a woman's life that is seriously affected by obesity and the related insulin resistance is "fertility." Obesity is a common risk factor for both PCOS and T2DM. Hyperinsulinemia secondary to insulin resistance is a stimulator of androgen secretion from the adrenal gland as well as the ovaries which in turn is responsible for anovulation. It is also found that obese women take longer time to conceive irrespective of their age and cyclic regularity. In fact, on a mean follow-up of 24 years, history of infertility and ovulation disorder was found to be independently associated with a higher lifetime risk of T2DM in women who did not have diabetes in reproductive years. On the other hand, uncontrolled diabetes is also associated with reduced fertility. Weight loss (by diet, exercise, and in some cases bariatric surgery) can improve the fertility of obese women by the return of spontaneous ovulation. Metformin is also found to be effective in improving the chances of successful conception in obese women with PCOS and T2DM. Weight loss with bariatric surgery has not only found to increase the fertility in obese women but also reduces the chances of gestational diabetes mellitus (GDM) and cesarean section in mothers. It also reduces the risk of macrosomia (without significantly increasing the risk of low birth weight) in the infant. Additionally, babies born to a mother after weight loss from bariatric surgery have lesser risk of developing obesity in adulthood.

Scenario 3

A 32-year-old lady known to have T2DM since 4 years presented at 10 weeks of unplanned pregnancy. She is on metformin and glimepiride tablets but monitoring and follow-up with physician are irregular. Current HbA1c is 8.9%.

In first place, preconception counseling should be an inevitable part of routine diabetes care for all women with diabetes and childbearing potential; so that glycemic control close to normal, ideally HbA1c less than 6.5% can be achieved to reduce the risk of congenital anomalies. In Indian culture, it is often a practice to overfeed pregnant women. Obese women with T2DM should be counseled for balanced diet and recommended weight gain during pregnancy which may be as low as 5–8 kg in contrast to 9–11 kg for normal weight women. In a planned pregnancy, oral antidiabetic agents should preferably be shifted to insulin, except in the setting of PCOS, where metformin can be safely used for ovulation induction. The safety of metformin in first trimester beyond ovulation induction remains unknown. Lessons from a systematic review that included more than 135,000 patients (80% women) found that bariatric surgery resulted in complete resolution of diabetes in 78% of patients and improvement in diabetic control in more than 86% of patients. Other medications like angiotensin-converting enzyme (ACE) inhibitors, angiotensin receptor blockers, or statins should be avoided in pregnancy and women with childbearing potential. From another perspective, addition of insulin before and during pregnancy may confer weight gain and adversely affect the lifetime metabolic risk.

Scenario 4

A 29-year-old obese woman currently 26 weeks pregnant detected with GDM.

Gestational diabetes poses medical, emotional, social as well as financial burden to not only the woman but also to the entire family. Gestational diabetes is significantly more prevalent in women with obesity. The medical management and intricacies are described elsewhere in this monograph. However, what is of equal importance and is often overlooked due to the joy of childbirth is the postpregnancy care of a mother with gestational diabetes. Gestational diabetes mellitus definitely seems to increase the probability of T2DM in a woman's lifetime but the exact risk is difficult to measure due mainly to heterogeneity in diagnostic criteria used. With the widespread acceptance of International Association for Diabetes in Pregnancy Study Group criteria, the prevalence of GDM is set to increase by two- to threefold. The most important predictor of future risk of diabetes in women with GDM is glycemic status at the time of diagnosis (results of oral glucose tolerance test) particularly the fasting blood glucose. Higher the glucose levels during an oral glucose tolerance test, higher the chances of conversion to T2DM in future. Other factors identified but found to be of less significance are body weight during the index pregnancy, lesser gestational age at diagnosis, family history of diabetes, and higher parity. While high postpregnancy weight is thought to increase the risk, breastfeeding (average 1 year following each delivery) and life-style measures to attain normal weight have been shown, to reduce the risk. Though it is often difficult to concentrate for caregivers, patients as well as the family on the future risk of T2DM to mother at this stage, but this time is an opportunity to educate and advise measures to prevent future complications.

Scenario 5

A 30-week-old female fetus in an obese and diabetic mother's womb.

Children of obese women are at a higher risk to develop obesity, diabetes mellitus, and cardiovascular diseases in their lifetime. Moreover, even after adjustment for prepregnancy BMI, maternal gestational diabetes significantly increases risk of overweight and obesity in the offspring. The relationship may reflect intrauterine fetal programming, genetic transmission, epigenetic alterations, impaired placental function, or shared environments such as postnatal diet and physical activity. Fetal hyperinsulinemia due to maternal hyperglycemia predisposes to increased adiposity, impaired glucose tolerance, hyperinsulinemia, and insulin resistance in the child. Treatment of gestational diabetes has shown to reduce the risk of the offspring to the level of an offspring born to a nondiabetic woman.

It is interesting to note that the effects of intrauterine fetal programming are also gender specific. That means the female fetus is affected differently than the male fetus. A study found that at 5 years of age, daughters of diabetic mothers had larger subscapular and triceps skinfold thickness and were more prone to develop impaired glucose tolerance and higher insulin concentrations compared to sons. It is also to be noted that such an effect on a female fetus initiates an intergenerational vicious cycle of metabolic abnormality. Finally, periconceptional weight loss potentially reverses these impacts of maternal obesity and GDM on the child and are of great importance for the prevention of future cardiometabolic risks in both. Thus, it is the best approach to break the intergenerational propagation of obesity and diabetes. However, it must weighed against the risk of maternal calorie restriction which also can adversely affect fetal programming and confer long-term metabolic risk, especially in areas where malnutrition is prevalent.

Scenario 6

A 62-year-old postmenopausal lady with diabetes, hypertension, dyslipidemia, and coronary artery disease.

With an increased expectancy of life, women are spending more time in the postmenopausal phase. Diabetes neutralises the cardiovascular protection provided by the female hormones prior to menopause. Obesity not only increases the risk of T2DM in postmenopausal women but also is an independent risk factor for musculoskeletal pain, osteoarthritis, depression, and cancers of reproductive organs such as endometrium, cervix, ovaries, and breast. There are disproportionately higher effects of T2DM on women. They not only have poorer glycemic control (reaching target HbA1c) but also have more symptoms of hyperglycemia than their male counterparts. Women with diabetes have a poorer prognosis after myocardial infarction and higher all-cause mortality, at the comparable HbA1c. Women with diabetes have an increased risk of hypertension and more severe type of dyslipidemia compared to men with diabetes. In many cohorts globally, women are less likely than men to receive lipid-lowering drugs, ACE inhibitors, calcium channel blockers, and aspirin for primary or secondary prevention of CAD (coronary artery disease), as well as lesser cardiac catheterization, percutaneous transluminal coronary angioplasty, and coronary artery bypass graft surgery during an acute coronary event. The scenario in India is likely to be graver due to cultural and social reasons affecting health access to women. It is very critical that recommendations for women with obesity and diabetes include exercise, constant advice to avoid weight gain, screening for CAD, daily aspirin when recommended, and aggressive treatment of acute coronary events. In women with obesity, antidiabetic medications with weight loss potential (glucagon-like peptide 1 analogs and sodium-glucose co-transporter 2 inhibitors) or at least those with weight neutrality (metformin, dipeptidyl peptidase-4 inhibitors) should be preferred if not contraindicated otherwise.

CONCLUSION

A woman's life is eventful with menstruation, pregnancy, breastfeeding, and menopause taking a toll on her overall health. Obesity is closely related to these events in reproductive life of a woman and increases the risk of T2DM. The biological advantage of coronary protection is lost at menopause as well as with occurrence of T2DM. Due to biological as well as various nonbiological factors women have a higher risk and a poorer outcome from treatment of T2DM. Special attention needs to be provided to prevent obesity and diabetes in women at every stage of their contact with medical care team throughout their life. Aggressive treatment of T2DM and obesity with diet, exercise, and medication as well as aggressive treatment of CAD is warranted. Bariatric surgery may be considered if the conventional approach fails.

SUGGESTED READINGS

1. Agrawal P, Gupta K, Mishra V, Agrawal S. Effects of sedentary lifestyle and dietary habits on body mass index change among adult women in India: findings from a follow-up study. Ecol Food Nutr. 2013;52(5):387-406.
2. Association AD. Management of diabetes in pregnancy. Diabetes Care. 2017;40 (Suppl 1):S114-9.
3. Bajaj S, Jawad F, Islam N, Mahtab H, Bhattarai J, Shrestha D, et al. South Asian women with diabetes: psychosocial challenges and management: Consensus statement. Indian J Endocrinol Metab. 2013;17(4):548-62.
4. Battista M-C, Hivert M-F, Duval K, Baillargeon J-P. Intergenerational cycle of obesity and diabetes: how can we reduce the burdens of these conditions on the health of future generations? Exp Diabetes Res. 2011;2011:596060.
5. Brown L, Clegg D. Central effects of estradiol in the regulation of adiposity. J Steroid Biochem Mol Biol. 2010;122(1-3):65-73.
6. Buchwald H, Estok R, Fahrbach K, Banel D, Jensen MD, Pories WJ, et al. Weight and type 2 diabetes after bariatric surgery: systematic review and meta-analysis. Am J Med. 2009;122(3):248-256.e5.
7. Chopra SM, Misra A, Gulati S, Gupta R. Overweight, obesity and related non-communicable diseases in Asian Indian girls and women. Eur J Clin Nutr. 2013;67(7):688-96.
8. Crawford MA, Mendoza-Vasconez AS, Larsen BA. Type II diabetes disparities in diverse women: the potential roles of body composition, diet, and physical activity. Womens Health Lond Engl. 2015;11(6):913-27.
9. Enzi G, Gasparo M, Biondetti PR, Fiore D, Semisa M, Zurlo F. Subcutaneous and visceral fat distribution according to sex, age, and overweight, evaluated by computed tomography. Am J Clin Nutr. 1986;44(6):739-46.
10. Geller DH, Pacaud D, Gordon CM, Misra M, of the Drug and Therapeutics Committee of the Pediatric Endocrine Society. State of the Art Review: Emerging Therapies: The Use of Insulin Sensitizers in the Treatment of Adolescents with Polycystic Ovary Syndrome (PCOS). Int J Pediatr Endocrinol. 2011;2011:9.
11. Guh DP, Zhang W, Bansback N, Amarsi Z, Birmingham CL, Anis AH. The incidence of co-morbidities related to obesity and overweight: A systematic review and meta-analysis. BMC Public Health. 2009;9:88.
12. Juutilainen A, Kortelainen S, Lehto S, Rönnemaa T, Pyörälä K, Laakso M. Gender difference in the impact of type 2 diabetes on coronary heart disease risk. Diabetes Care. 2004;27(12):2898-904.
13. Kalra S, Unnikrishnan AG. Obesity in India: The weight of the nation. J Med Nutr Nutraceuticals. 2012;1(1):37.
14. Kim C, Halter JB. Endogenous sex hormones, metabolic syndrome, and diabetes in men and women. Curr Cardiol Rep. 2014;16(4):467.
15. Kim SY, Sharma AJ, Callaghan WM. Gestational diabetes and childhood obesity: what is the link? Curr Opin Obstet Gynecol. 2012;24(6):376-81.
16. Kupelian V, Page ST, Araujo AB, Travison TG, Bremner WJ, McKinlay JB. Low sex hormone-binding globulin, total testosterone, and symptomatic androgen deficiency are associated with development of the metabolic syndrome in nonobese men. J Clin Endocrinol Metab. 2006;91(3):843-50.
17. Legato MJ, Gelzer A, Goland R, Ebner SA, Rajan S, Villagra V, et al. Gender-specific care of the patient with diabetes: review and recommendations. Gend Med. 2006;3(2):131-58.
18. National Family Health Survey. [online] Available from: http://rchiips.org/nfhs/sub_report.shtml [Accessed April, 2017].

19. Noctor E, Dunne FP. Type 2 diabetes after gestational diabetes: the influence of changing diagnostic criteria. World J Diabetes. 2015;6(2):234-44.
20. Phillips PJ. Women, coronary artery disease and diabetes. Aust Fam Physician. 2008;37(6):441-2.
21. Ranjani H, Sonya J, Anjana RM, Mohan V. Prevalence of glucose intolerance among children and adolescents in urban South India (ORANGE-2). Diabetes Technol Ther. 2013;15(1):13-9.
22. Reinehr T. Type 2 diabetes mellitus in children and adolescents. World J Diabetes. 2013;4(6):270-81.
23. Roche MM, Wang PP. Sex differences in all-cause and cardiovascular mortality, hospitalization for individuals with and without diabetes, and patients with diabetes diagnosed early and late. Diabetes Care. 2013;36(9):2582-90.
24. Smith J, Cianflone K, Biron S, Hould FS, Lebel S, Marceau S, et al. Effects of maternal surgical weight loss in mothers on intergenerational transmission of obesity. J Clin Endocrinol Metab. 2009;94(11):4275-83.
25. Tobias DK, Gaskins AJ, Missmer SA, Hu FB, Manson JE, Buck Louis GM, et al. History of infertility and risk of type 2 diabetes mellitus: a prospective cohort study. Diabetologia. 2015;58(4):707-15.
26. van der Steeg JW, Steures P, Eijkemans MJC, Habbema JDF, Hompes PG, Burggraaff JM, et al. Obesity affects spontaneous pregnancy chances in subfertile, ovulatory women. Hum Reprod Oxf Engl. 2008;23(2):324-8.
27. Wasalathanthri S. Attenuating type 2 diabetes with postpartum interventions following gestational diabetes mellitus. World J Diabetes. 2015;6(4):648-53.

9

CHAPTER

Dyslipidemia and Hypertension

Anuj Maheshwari, Brij M Makkar

INTRODUCTION

Across the globe, cardiovascular disease (CVD) is considered as men's problem. However, it is top killer in women in Europe causing 51% death of those suffering with this, while in India, cardiovascular (CV) risk accounts for 15% of global burden. About 3 in 5 women in India keep on higher risk of CVD at early age of 35 years. Largest percentage of women in India remains on CV risk between the age group of 35 and 44 years that includes 69% housewives which is not much different than percentage of working women on CV risk i.e., 67%. It seems Indian women lose their normal female protection from CVD very early.

Women may present with a variety of symptoms to various specialists but rarely evaluated for syndrome and associated illnesses. Mostly, they are treated for presenting complaint only. Multidisciplinary healthcare system actually fails to deliver here in case of women because of tubular vision of healthcare providers. In India, women are usually deprived of multidisciplinary healthcare system. Largely, they are treated by one healthcare provider of same gender for all their problems, irrespective of specialty. Diabetic women have 50% greater risk of CVD. Women with diabetes do not enjoy gender specific female protection from CVD. They are three times more likely to die of coronary heart disease (CHD) as compared to those without diabetes.

DIABETES IN WOMEN—THE CHALLENGES

According to data published in 2013, over 371 million individuals across the world have diabetes and approximately half of these are women. With increasing lifespan, proportion of females at more risk of diabetes is also rising. The World Health Organization reports that 55% of diabetes-related deaths occur in women, and these are primarily due to risk of CVD.

Women with diabetes carry a higher burden of multiple CV risk factors, including hypertension and dyslipidemia. A gender-based analysis from the INTERHEART study found that a number of risk factors (including hypertension, diabetes, high alcohol intake, and low physical activity) were carrying more strong relationship in women than in men, consequently raising the risk of myocardial infarction (MI) in this high-risk population. In this global case-control study which included 27,098 participants from 52 countries, 6,787 of those were women, the median age of first acute MI was higher in women than men (65 vs. 56 years; $p < 0.0001$). Hypertension and diabetes (in addition to physical activity and moderate alcohol use) have been found to have stronger association with occurrence of MI among women than men.

Similarly, in another study on dyslipidemia, increased low-density lipoprotein cholesterol (LDL-C) levels were related to CVD in both the genders, but low high-density lipoproteins cholesterol (HDL-C) and increased triglyceride levels have been seen to be more strongly related to CVD in women than in men, with 70% higher risk in women compared with 30% risk in men.

This clustering of risk factors including increased blood glucose, hypertension and cholesterol abnormalities (in addition to obesity) is often a result of insulin resistance, an aspect often attributed to hormonal regulation by estrogen in women.

Dyslipidemia and Hypertension in Gestational Diabetes Mellitus Carries a Long-term Risk

There is a physiological rise in total cholesterol, triglycerides, and lipoproteins in normal pregnancy, and these spikes are attributed to the pregnancy hormones, including human chorionic gonadotropin hormone, β-estradiol, insulin, and progesterone.

However, abnormally elevated triglycerides, total cholesterol, and LDL-C during pregnancy are also associated with pregnancy-related hypertension.Studies suggest that women carrying low HDL-C and high triglycerides level before conception have higher chance of preeclampsia and/or gestational diabetes.

Additionally, women who experience hypertensive disorder in pregnancy are diagnosed with hypertension more often and early in life as opposed to women who do not experience this complication. These women are also at higher risk of CVD, primarily because of hypertension. Similarly, women with gestational diabetes are likely to be detected with type 2 diabetes mellitus (T2DM) and hypertension much earlier in life.

Dyslipidemia in Women

Hormonal changes occurring throughout lifetime of women like at puberty, menarche, pregnancy, and menopause alter serum lipoprotein level. At the time of birth, and throughout childhood, serum cholesterol levels are not different between boys and girls; however, boys have a lesser size of LDL particle as compared with girls. The LDL-C levels are likely to rise in both the genders after 20 years of age, but do so more rapidly in men.

Similarly, boys and girls differ in the HDL particle size, with boys and male adolescents having smaller HDL particle size as compared with females. In boys the size of HDL particle decreases with advancement of age while in girls it remains stable. These lipoprotein differences between the genders beginning in childhood usually offer CV protection in premenopausal women.

Use of oral contraceptive pills (OCPs) brings the changes in level of lipoproteins depending upon ratio of estrogen and progesterone present in them. The estrogen component present in OCPs causes increase in HDL-C, HDL2, and triglyceride levels and decrease in LDL-C levels. The progesterone component is supposed to have exactly opposite effect on lipoprotein than that of estrogen.

It is well established that postmenopausal women are likely to have significantly different lipid profiles as compared with premenopausal women. Menopausal transition leads to various lipoprotein changes including increased levels of LDL-C, total cholesterol, and apolipoprotein B as compared with those occurring before menopause. There is an additional transition of LDL particles to more atherogenic smaller and denser particles. Total HDL-C and HDL2 also decrease in postmenopausal women.

The use of unopposed estrogen as hormone replacement therapy (HRT) is associated with significantly higher HDL-C and HDL2 and lower LDL-C as compared with premenopausal women. However, combination HRT is likely to negate the rise in HDL occurring with estrogen monotherapy.

In the Postmenopausal Estrogen and Progesterone Interventions trial, it has been seen that combination HRT having progesterone also caused a significantly lesser rise in HDL-C and triglycerides as compared with estrogen-only HRT.

Clinical Consequences of Dyslipidemia

The Lipid Research Clinics' Follow-up Study found HDL-C and triglycerides strong predictors of CV mortality while LDL-C and total cholesterol as poor predictors after analyzing various lipid abnormalities in 1,405 females between 50 and 69 years of age. The HDL-C level less than 50 mg/dL posed 30% more risk for CV mortality while those with triglyceride level 200–399 mg/dL had 65% higher risk.

High triglyceride levels have been found to be associated with approximately 30% higher CHD risk in men while 75% higher risk in females in a meta-analysis of 17 population-based studies which have prospectively evaluated this association of triglyceride with CV risks. Further, young females having predominantly high level of small atherogenic LDL-C particles as well as elevated lipoprotein(a) had a raised risk of a CV event.

Approach to Management of Dyslipidemia in Women

It has been widely recommended that women should undergo statin therapy for primary prevention after the assessment of risk as per the guideline recommendations while those with established atherosclerosis should be treated with a statin. Statin therapy is very well shown to be efficacious in women.

The Justification for the Use of Statins in Prevention: An Intervention Trial Evaluating Rosuvastatin (JUPITER) which included 6,801 women 60 years or more of age and 11,001 men 50 years or more of age with high-sensitivity C-reactive protein 2 mg/L or more and LDL-C <130 mg/dL randomized to rosuvastatin versus placebo, demonstrated that rosuvastatin used in primary prevention reduced CV events in women with equally good relative risk reduction as in men. Meta-analysis of primary prevention trials of statin has also supported it.

Meta-analysis of placebo-controlled studies of statin for primary prevention in females in which statin has been used primarily to know gender-specific outcomes in most of the women or all (20,147 women; >276 CVD events; mean age, 63–69 years) has been done. Absolute CV mortality per 100 person per years in women in JUPITER was found lesser than for men after giving rosuvastatin and placebo (women—0.57 and 1.04, respectively; men—0.88 and 1.54, respectively) although relative risk reduction was similar in women (hazard ratio, 0.54; 95% confidence interval (CI), 0.37–0.80; p = 0.002) and men (hazard ratio, 0.58; 95% Cl, 0.45–0.73; p <0.001). Revascularization or unstable angina have been significantly reduced in women with reduction in other components of primary end point also, though nonsignificant statistically. A significant one-third fall in primary CVD events with statin (relative risk, 0.63; 95% Cl, 0.49–0.82; p <0.001; P for heterogeneity = 0.56) has been shown in a meta-analysis of 13,154 women (240 CVD events; 216 total deaths) in exclusively primary prevention trials but with only small nonsignificant reduction in total mortality (relative risk, 0.78; 95% Cl, 0.53–1.15; p = 0.21; p for heterogeneity = 0.20). Results were comparable in trials where statin was used predominantly but not exclusively for primary prevention.

Hypertension in Women

High blood pressure is significant, modifiable risk factor for CV mortality and morbidity which is widely prevalent too, in both the sexes. Usually it is higher in men irrespective of age but more women are having hypertension after 65 years of age which is more severe also as compared to men. Severity and prevalence both increases in women with age. Worldwide prevalence is expected to increase more in women, i.e.,13%

as compared with men which is 9% between the year 2000 and 2025. Around 483.5 million women had hypertension in the year 2000 which is expected to rise 793.3 million in 2025.

Role of Menopause in Hypertension in Women

Epidemiological studies suggest that the incidence of hypertension increases in postmenopausal women as compared with premenopausal women. Estrogen's deficiency can induce endothelial dysfunction and increased body mass index causing hypertension in this phase of life.

As with dyslipidemia, oral contraceptives also raise the risk of hypertension. In women suffering from hypertension, discontinuation of combined oral contraceptive pills may lower blood pressure. Poorly controlled hypertension can cause threefold rise in risk of MI and strokes but risk of hemorrhagic stroke may go up 15-fold. Progestogen only contraceptives may be more useful in women carrying multiple CV risk factors.

The Insulin-resistance Syndrome in Women

As discussed earlier, features of the metabolic syndrome (insulin resistance, abdominal obesity, and dyslipidemia) commonly emerge with the estrogen decline experienced during menopause. It is well known that estrogen is involved in a number of mechanisms which regulate body fat distribution and glucose and lipid metabolism. However, there is also a growing population of young women who exhibit the metabolic syndrome. In addition, gestational diabetes mellitus raises the risk of the syndrome in the long term. This underscores the need to further examine sex-specific mechanisms and tailored therapies to ameliorate long-term cardiometabolic risk in these susceptible women.

Long-term Implications

Women with T2DM compared with men with T2DM are at greater risk of a CV event. A 5-year follow-up study showed that women were eight times more likely than men to experience a composite endpoint of death, acute MI, unstable angina, coronary intervention, heart failure, cerebral ischemic stroke or transient ischemic attack, or peripheral artery disease.

Data over 6–8 years from the Nurses' Health Study and Health Professionals Follow-up Study show that the relative risk of CHD in individuals with the metabolic syndrome compared with those without the metabolic syndrome was higher in women than in men (relative risk, 3.01 vs. 1.62, respectively; $p = 0.03$).

The worse outcomes in women have been attributed primarily to dyslipidemia and obesity. Postprandial hyperglycemia and hypertension also worsen outcomes.

SUGGESTED READINGS

1. Anand SS, Islam S, Rosengren A, et al. Risk factors for myocardial infarction in women and men: insights from the INTERHEART study. Eur Heart J. 2008;29:932-40.
2. Bajaj S, Jawad F, Islam N, et al. South Asian women with diabetes: Psychosocial challenges and management: Consensus statement. Indian J Endocrinol Metab. 2013;17:548-62.
3. Bass KM, Newschaffer CJ, Klag MJ, et al. Plasma lipoprotein levels as predictors of cardiovascular death in women. Arch Intern Med. 1993;153(19):2209-16.
4. Baumfield Y, Novack L, Wiznitzer A, et al. Pre-conception dyslipidemia is associated with development of preeclampsia and gestational diabetes mellitus. PLoS One. 2015;10(10): e0139164.
5. Heida KY, Franx A, van Rijn BB, et al. Earlier age of onset of chronic hypertension and type 2 diabetes mellitus after a hypertensive disorder of pregnancy or gestational diabetes mellitus. Hypertension. 2015;66(6):1116-22.
6. Hokanson JE, Austin MA. Plasma triglyceride level is a risk factor for cardiovascular disease independent of high-density lipoprotein cholesterol level: a meta-analysis of population-based prospective studies. J Cardiovasc Risk. 1996;3(2):213-9.
7. Hokansson JE, Austin MA. Plasma triglyceride level is a risk factor for cardiovascular disease independent of high-density lipoprotein cholesterol level: a meta-analysis of population based prospective studies. J Cardiovasc Risk. 1996;3:213-9.
8. Kamigaki AS, Siscovick DS, Schwartz SM, et al. Low density lipoprotein particle size and risk of early-onset myocardial infarction in women. Am J Epidemiol. 2001;153(10):939-45.
9. Kaminski P, Szpotanska-Sikorska M, Wielgos M. Cardiovascular risk and the use of oral contraceptives. Neuro Endocrinol Lett. 2013;34(7):587-9.
10. Meade TW. Randomised comparison of oestrogen versus oestrogen plus progestogen hormone replacement therapy in women with hysterectomy. Medical Research Council's General Practice Research Framework. BMJ. 1996;312(7029):473-8.
11. Modena MG. Hypertension in postmenopausal women: how to approach hypertension in menopause. High Blood Press Cardiovasc Prev. 2014;21(3):201-4.
12. Mora S, Glynn RJ, Hsia J, et al. Statins for the primary prevention of cardiovascular events in women with elevated high-sensitivity C-reactive protein or dyslipidemia: results from the Justification for the Use of Statins in Prevention: An Intervention Trial Evaluating Rosuvastatin (JUPITER) and meta-analysis of women from primary prevention trials. Circulation. 2010;121(9):1069-77.
13. Norhammar A, Schenck-Gustafsson K. Type 2 diabetes and cardiovascular disease in women. Diabetologia. 2013;56:1-9.
14. Phan BAP, Toth PP. Dyslipidemia in women: etiology and management. Int J Womens Health. 2014;6:185-94.
15. Pimenta E. Hypertension in women. Hypertens Res. 2012;35:148-52.
16. Pischon T, Hu FB, Rexrode KM, et al. Inflammation, the metabolic syndrome, and risk of coronary heart disease in women and men. Atherosclerosis. 2008;197(1):392.
17. Pradhan AD. Sex differences in the metabolic syndrome: implications for cardiovascular health in women. Clin Chem. 2014;60(1): 44-52.
18. Pradhan AD. Sex differences in the metabolic syndrome: implications for cardiovascular health in women. Clin Chem. 2014;60(1):44-52.
19. Zandbergen AA, Sijbrands EJ, Lamberts SW, et al. Normotensive women with type 2 diabetes and microalbuminuria are at high risk for macrovascular disease. Diabetes Care. 2006;29(8):1851-5.

10

CHAPTER

Vitamin D

Gagan Priya, Rajat Gupta

INTRODUCTION

Vitamin D regulates calcium metabolism and bone mineralization and its deficiency is traditionally associated with rickets, osteomalacia, muscle weakness, reduced bone density, and risk of fractures. There has been immense interest in the noncalcitropic functions of vitamin D as most cells express the vitamin D receptor (VDR) and can also produce the biologically active form of vitamin D [$1,25(OH)_2D$] for paracrine functions. Vitamin D regulates a multitude of biological functions—cell differentiation, angiogenesis, apoptosis, immunomodulation, neuroprotection, glucose metabolism, and cardiovascular health.

Vitamin D deficiency (VDD) is a global public health problem affecting all age groups, especially females. Lack of sunlight exposure, extremes of latitude, winter season, conservative clothing, dark skin pigmentation, aging, sunscreens, air pollution, obesity, and lack of food fortification are some factors that affect vitamin D status. In a recent report of global health trends, VDD (<20 ng/mL) was reported in 91% adolescent females, 66% adults, 91% elderly, and 96% pregnant or lactating women in India. About 62% elderly and 60% pregnant or lactating women had 25(OH)D levels less than 12 ng/mL.

VITAMIN D AND IMMUNOMODULATION

Vitamin D has immunomodulatory and anti-inflammatory properties. $1,25(OH)_2D$ modulates innate immune response by downregulating the expression of monocyte toll-like receptor 2 (TLR2) and TLR4, thus suppressing inflammatory response. It inhibits the maturation of dendritic cells and their capacity to present antigens to T-cells and increases their apoptosis.

It suppresses the expression of major histocompatibility complex-II and costimulatory molecules and reduces immunogenicity while promoting immune tolerance.

Vitamin D also has an inhibitory effect on adaptive immunity and promotes a shift from Th1 to Th2 cell function. It suppresses proinflammatory Th1 cytokines [interleukin-2 (IL-2), IL-6, interferon-γ, and tumor necrosis factor-β] and enhances anti-inflammatory Th2 cytokines (IL-2, IL-10, and transforming growth factor-β1). 1,25$(OH)_2$D also inhibits the proliferation of B-cells, inhibits immunoglobulin production, and induces their apoptosis.

EFFECTS OF VITAMIN D ON GLUCOSE HOMEOSTASIS

Figure 1 illustrates the role of vitamin D in glucose homeostasis.

Effects on Pancreatic Function

Vitamin D promotes pancreatic β-cell function via direct and indirect actions:

- Direct genomic action: Binds to VDR and regulates transcription of target genes via vitamin D responsive elements. Thus, it enhances insulin synthesis and secretion and promotes β-cell survival by reducing cytokine-induced apoptosis
- Indirect rapid action: Regulates calbindin (a cytosolic Ca-binding protein in β-cells) and intracellular calcium. Hence, it acts as a modulator of depolarization-stimulated insulin release.

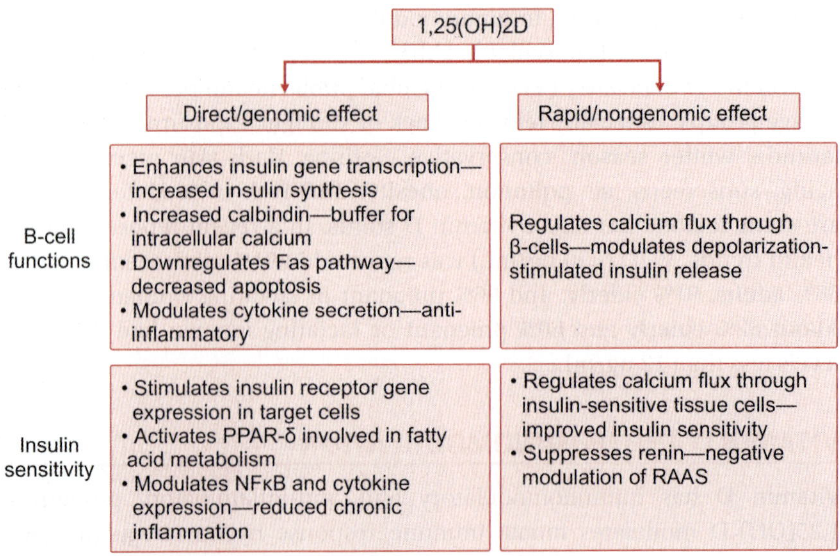

1,25(OH)2D, 1,25-dihydroxyvitamin D; PPAR, peroxisome proliferator-activated receptor; NF, nuclear factor; RAAS, renin-angiotensin-aldosterone system.

FIG. 1: Role of vitamin D in glucose homeostasis

Effects on Insulin Sensitivity

Vitamin D directly stimulates the expression of insulin receptors in insulin-responsive tissues (skeletal muscle and adipose tissue) and also activates the peroxisome proliferator-activated receptor delta that regulates fatty acid metabolism. An indirect effect on insulin sensitivity may be mediated via regulation of intracellular calcium concentration within a narrow range. Further, its immunomodulatory effects may lead to reduced chronic inflammation and improved insulin sensitivity. Vitamin D also suppresses renin formation and could be a negative regulator of renin-angiotensin-aldosterone system (RAAS).

In addition, low vitamin D may induce secondary hyperparathyroidism. Raised parathyroid hormone causes a paradoxical increase in intracellular calcium (calcium paradox), which inhibits insulin synthesis and secretion in β-cells and induces insulin resistance in target cells.

VITAMIN D AND TYPE 1 DIABETES MELLITUS

Type 1 diabetes mellitus (T1DM) is caused by progressive autoimmune destruction of pancreatic islets and is characterized by chronic inflammatory insulitis. Studies have shown an association between VDD and risk of T1DM. Observational studies suggest an inverse correlation between incidence of T1DM and sunlight exposure. Vitamin D has a potential role in prevention and progression of T1DM due to its immunomodulatory and anti-inflammatory effects.

High doses of $1,25(OH)_2D$ suppressed insulitis and development of hyperglycemia in animal models of T1DM nonobese diabetic mice. Structural analogs of $1,25(OH)_2D$ (14-epivitamin D_3 analog TX527) are being investigated to avoid the risk of hypercalcemia and tissue calcification associated with high dose calcitriol. Vitamin D analogs have been shown to halt the progression of T1DM even after the initiation of autoimmune attack.

Does Vitamin D Supplementation Reduce the Risk of Type 1 Diabetes Mellitus or Its Progression?

Small interventional studies suggested that risk of T1DM may be decreased by vitamin D supplementation of mothers in the third trimester of pregnancy or of infants in the first year of life. The European Diabetes (EURODIAB) study reported a 33% risk reduction of T1DM in children who received vitamin D supplementation in early life. A recent meta-analysis of eight studies suggested a 29% risk reduction (odds ratio 0.71, 95% confidence interval 0.51–0.98) in infants supplemented with vitamin D but effect of maternal vitamin D intake of risk of T1DM in offspring was not significant. No large prospective randomized control studies are yet available to support a definitive role of vitamin D in T1DM prevention. Vitamin D analogs are being investigated for their role in reducing rejection rates following islet cell transplantation.

VITAMIN D AND TYPE 2 DIABETES MELLITUS

Vitamin D deficiency has been associated with obesity, metabolic syndrome, type 2 diabetes mellitus (T2DM), hypertension, atherosclerosis, coronary artery disease, and stroke. Obesity results in sequestration of vitamin D in adipose tissue with decreased availability of active vitamin D in serum. Dietary habits, sedentary lifestyle, renal impairment, and polymorphism of vitamin D binding protein may further predispose to VDD.

National Health and Nutrition Examination Survey III demonstrated a positive relationship of serum 25(OH)D levels with insulin sensitivity and an inverse relationship with metabolic syndrome, in all racial and ethnic groups. In a 20-year prospective cohort of 83,779 women in the Nurses' Health Study, a combined daily intake of more than 1,200 mg calcium and more than 800 IU vitamin D was associated with a 33% lower risk [risk ratio (RR) 0.67, 0.49–0.90] of T2DM, compared to a daily intake of less than 600 mg calcium and less than 400 IU vitamin D. In the Women's Health Study involving a large cohort of postmenopausal women, higher calcium intake was associated with lower prevalence of metabolic syndrome. There was a small but insignificant association with higher vitamin D intake. A meta-analysis of 21 prospective studies showed an inverse and significant association (RR 0.62, 0.54–0.70) between 25(OH)D levels and risk of T2DM in diverse populations. People with T2DM and prediabetes had low vitamin D levels than people with normal glucose tolerance in several cross-sectional studies.

Does Vitamin D Supplementation Improve Glucose Control or Prevent Diabetes?

Calcitriol has been shown to improve hyperglycemia in animal models of T2DM with improvement in insulin secretion. Small intervention studies have variably reported improvements in insulin secretion and glycemic control with vitamin D. However, a systematic review of 35 randomized controlled trials (RCTs) showed no effect of vitamin D supplementation on progression to new diabetes and on insulin resistance (HOMA-IR), insulin secretion (HOMA-β), fasting glucose or HbA1c in those with T2DM. In another recent meta-analysis of 21 RCTs, there was no effect on HbA1c, but a significant effect was seen on fasting glucose in those with HbA1c greater than 8%. Similarly, no effect has been found on weight, fat mass, waist circumference, or blood pressure. Well-designed, long-term intervention trials are needed to address the potential role of vitamin D in T2DM.

VITAMIN D AND DIABETIC COMPLICATIONS

Vitamin D deficiency has been associated with low bone density and/or quality, osteomalacia, muscle weakness, and increased risk of falls in postmenopausal women. The bone mineral density (BMD) has been reported to be normal, slightly higher, or lower in postmenopausal women with T2DM, but the fracture risk is high and has been attributed to poor bone quality. In a study from South India, BMD at femoral neck and lumbar spine was significantly lower in women with T2DM compared to controls. Vitamin D supplementation in elderly women reduces the risk of osteoporotic fractures and is routinely advisable.

Vitamin D deficiency is associated with hypertension and cardiovascular risk, though it may be a consequence, rather than a cause of cardiovascular disease. Evidence so far does not indicate a beneficial effect of vitamin D supplementation on risk of myocardial infarction, stroke, or cardiovascular mortality. Vitamin D deficiency has also been linked to microvascular complications. Observation studies have demonstrated a significant link between VDD and diabetic polyneuropathy and the odds ratio for diabetic polyneuropathy was 2.68 (95% CI 1.67–4.30) in those with VDD. It may exacerbate symptoms of painful diabetic neuropathy and vitamin D may have analgesic as well neuroprotective benefits. However, intervention trials in this regard are lacking. Vitamin D has also been postulated to have nephroprotective effects. A vitamin D analog (paracalcitriol) significantly lowered blood pressure and albuminuria in combination with RAAS inhibition. A recent review suggested that while there is a higher risk of diabetic nephropathy in VDD patients, supplementation did not suggest causality. Patients with chronic kidney disease have deficiency of both 25(OH)D and 1,25$(OH)_2$D and may need supplementation of both vitamin D and activated vitamin D (calcitriol). Caution is needed as high doses may be associated with vascular calcification. The association with diabetic retinopathy is even weaker.

VITAMIN D AND GESTATIONAL DIABETES

Vitamin D receptor and 1α-hydroxylase are expressed in pituitary, ovary, uterus, and placenta, and 1,25$(OH)_2D_3$ may have a role in modulating ovarian function. An inverse relationship exists between serum 25(OH)D levels and insulin resistance, waist hip ratio, body mass index, serum testosterone, and dehydroepiandrosterone sulfate levels in women with polycystic ovarian syndrome (PCOS).

During pregnancy, maternal vitamin D is required for appropriate fetal development. Vitamin D deficiency in pregnant women has been associated with preterm births, small-for-gestational age, preeclampsia, gestational diabetes mellitus (GDM), and maternal and neonatal infections. Higher vitamin D levels have been associated with less insulin resistance in pregnancy. Women with VDD had a significantly increased risk of GDM in a recent meta-analysis. However, in a study from India, there was no relation between 25(OH)D levels in second trimester and incidence of GDM.

Vitamin D also has a possible role in "fetal programing" by influencing genomic programing of fetal development and later risk of chronic diseases such as asthma, metabolic syndrome, T1DM, and schizophrenia.

Does Vitamin D Supplementation in Pregnancy Reduce the Risk of Gestational Diabetes Mellitus or Adverse Pregnancy Outcomes?

Small interventional studies suggest that vitamin D may improve insulin sensitivity and fasting glucose in pregnancy. A recent Cochrane review of 15 trials found a beneficial effect of vitamin D supplementation on risk of preeclampsia, preterm birth and low birth weight but no benefit on risk of GDM. Vitamin D supplements also were associated with greater infant length and head circumference at birth. Randomized controlled trials are needed to explore the potential protective role of vitamin D in development of GDM and its health outcomes in both mother and neonate.

There is limited evidence of safety of vitamin D supplementation during pregnancy—one study suggests that up to 4,000 IU/day did not cause hypercalcemia or hypercalciuria. High doses of vitamin D in pregnancy may increase risk for teratogenesis, growth restriction, delayed ossification, and craniofacial hypoplasia.

MANAGEMENT OF VITAMIN D DEFICIENCY

Serum 25(OH)D concentration is used as an indicator of overall vitamin D status in an individual. Vitamin D deficiency is defined as serum 25(OH)D less than or equal to 20 ng/mL. Table 1 depicts the

Table 1: Recommended daily intake of vitamin D

Age group	Institute of Medicine recommendation (IU)	Endocrine Society recommendation (IU)	Upper tolerable limit (IU)
0–1 year	400	400–1,000	2,000
1–18 years	600	600–1,000	4,000
19–70 years	600	1,500–2,000	10,000
>70 years	800	1,500–2,000	10,000
Pregnancy/lactation	600	1,500–2,000	10,000

Note: Obese, those on concomitant drugs (glucocorticoids, anticonvulsants, antifungals, antiretroviral drugs), or those with malabsorption require at 2–3 times more vitamin D to meet their requirements.

Source: Adapted from Endocrine Society Practice Guidelines 2011.

Table 2: Treatment of vitamin D deficiency		
Age group	**Dose for correction of vitamin D deficiency**	**Maintenance dose**
0–1 year	2,000 IU/day or 50,000 IU/week for 6 weeks	400–1,000 IU/day
1–18 years	2,000 IU/day or 50,000 IU/week for 6 weeks	600–1,000 IU/day
Adults	6,000 IU/day or 50,000 IU/week for 8 weeks	1,500–2,000 IU/day

Note: Target to achieve and sustain 25(OH)D levels >30 ng/mL. Obese, those on concomitant drugs (glucocorticoids, anticonvulsants, antifungals, antiretroviral drugs) or malabsorption require at 2–3 times more vitamin D to meet their requirements.

Source: Adapted from Endocrine Society Practice Guidelines 2011.

Recommended Dietary Intake of vitamin D (Endocrine Society Clinical Practice Guidelines 2011). While routine vitamin D measurement is not recommended, it is advisable in those at high risk of VDD.

In the absence of a clear evidence of noncalcemic benefits, routine vitamin D supplementation is not recommended to improve glycemic control in diabetes or for diabetes prevention but has a role in fall prevention in postmenopausal women. However, correction of established VDD and maintenance of adequate intake is advisable. For the correction of VDD, various dosing regimens from single intramuscular high dose (3-6 lakh IU) to weekly or daily administration have been used. Both vitamin D3 and D2 can be used, though some studies suggest greater efficacy of vitamin D3. One simple suggested protocol for various age groups is shown in table 2 (Endocrine Society Clinical Practice Guidelines 2011).

Currently, guidelines do not recommend routine serum 25(OH)D measurement in pregnant women but screening may be considered in those at high risk. There is insufficient evidence to assess the benefits or risks of vitamin D supplementation during pregnancy on maternal and fetal outcomes. In case of documented VDD, up to 1,000 IU/day may be needed to maintain 25(OH)D levels more than 20 ng/mL in pregnant women.

CONCLUSION

Due to its immunomodulatory and anti-inflammatory effects, vitamin D may help retard the progression to T1DM in genetically susceptible individuals. Vitamin D also regulates insulin secretion and insulin sensitivity and an inverse relationship between T2DM or GDM and vitamin D has been seen in cross-sectional and prospective studies. There is paucity of well-designed intervention trials to establish causality or benefits of vitamin D supplementation beyond bone and muscle health. However, there is a high prevalence of VDD among women, its treatment is simple and may offer additional health benefits in diabetes.

SUGGESTED READINGS

1. De-Regil LM, Palacios C, Lombardo LK, et al. Vitamin D supplementation for women during pregnancy. Cochrane Database Syst Rev. 2012;(2):CD008873.
2. Farrant HJ, Krishnaveni GV, Hill JC, et al. Vitamin D insufficiency is common in Indian mothers but is not associated with gestational diabetes or variation in newborn size. Eur J Clin Nutr. 2009;63(5):646-52.
3. Harinarayan CV. Vitamin D and diabetes mellitus. Hormones. 2014;13(2):163-81.
4. Holick MF, Binkley NC, Bischoff-Ferrari HA, et al. Evaluation, treatment, and prevention of vitamin D deficiency: an endocrine society clinical practice guideline. J Clin Endocrinol Metab. 2011;96(7):1911-30.
5. Dong JY1, Zhang WG, Chen JJ, et al. Vitamin D intake and risk of type 1 Diabetes: A meta-analysis of observational studies. Nutrients. 2013;5(9):3551-62.
6. Krul-Poel YHM, M ter Wee M, Lips P, et al. The effect of vitamin D supplementation on glycemic control in patients with type 2 diabetes mellitus: a systematic review and meta-analysis. Eur J Endocrinol. 2017;176:R1-14.
7. Liu S1, Song Y, Ford ES, et al. Dietary calcium, vitamin D, and the prevalence of metabolic syndrome in middle-aged and older U.S. women. Diabetes Care. 2005;28(12):2926-32.
8. Majumdar V, Nagaraja D, Christopher R. Vitamin D status and metabolic syndrome in Asian Indians. Int J Obes. 2011;35(8):1131-4.
9. Marwaha RK, Tandon N, Chopra S, et al. Vitamin D status in pregnant Indian women across trimesters and different seasons and its correlation with neonatal serum 25-hydroxyvitamin D levels. Br J Nutr. 2011;106(9):1383-9.
10. Marwaha RK, Tandon N, Garg MK, et al. Vitamin D status in healthy Indians aged 50 years and above. J Assoc Physicians India. 2011;59:706-9.
11. Palacios C, Gonzalez L. Is vitamin D deficiency a major global public health problem? J Steroid Biochem Mol Biol. 2014;144 Pt A:138-45.
12. Pittas AG, Dawson-Hughes B, Li T, et al. Vitamin D and calcium intake in relation to type 2 diabetes in women. Diabetes Care. 2006;29(3):650-6.
13. Pratheesh GM, Thabah MM, Zachariah B, et al. Decreased bone mineral density at the femoral neck and lumbar spine in South Indian patients with Type 2 Diabetes. J Clin Diagn Res. 2015;9(9):OC08-12.
14. Puri S, Marwaha RK, Agarwal N, et al. Vitamin D status of apparently healthy schoolgirls from two different socioeconomic strata in Delhi: relation to nutrition and lifestyle. Br J Nutr. 2008;99(4):876-82.
15. Seida JC, Mitri J, Colmers IN, et al. Clinical review: Effect of vitamin D3 supplementation on improving glucose homeostasis and preventing diabetes: a systematic review and meta-analysis. J Clin Endocrinol Metab. 2014;99(10):3551-60.
16. Song Y, Wang L, Pittas AG, et al. Blood 25-hydroxy vitamin D levels and incident type 2 diabetes: a meta-analysis of prospective studies. Diabetes Care. 2013;36(5):1422-8.
17. Zhang M Xi, Pan GT, Guo JF, et al. Vitamin D deficiency increases the risk of gestational diabetes mellitus: a meta-analysis of observational studies. Nutrients. 2015;7(10):8366-75.

11
CHAPTER

Cardiovascular Disease

Mala Dharmalingam, Ganavi YP

INTRODUCTION

One of the major causes of mortality in India is cardiovascular diseases (CVDs). The recent advances in the field of cardiovascular medicine are the differences in the pathophysiological factors between men and women. To understand these is of crucial importance for the diagnosis and treatment and to develop new gender-specific management protocols.

EPIDEMIOLOGY

Cardiovascular diseases occur a decade earlier and in the most productive period of life in Indians. In men and women, ischemic heart disease, stroke, and other CVDs account for 21, 11, and 11% of the cases and 23, 18, and 15%, respectively. It has been stated that 1 in 3 adult women have some form of CVD. The life expectancy in females is longer than males; as a result, there has been a rising trend of loss of disability-adjusted life years in women. This could also be explained by the fact that there is an increase in myocardial infarction in older women with a concomitant decrease in men.

PATHOLOGY/SEX-RELATED CARDIOVASCULAR DISEASE RISK FACTORS

There are traditional cardiovascular risk factors, which determine progression to CVD in men and women, but a few gender differences have been illustrated (Box 1).

Women have a higher sympathetic inhibition, cardiac vagal tone, heart rate variability, and lower susceptibility to arrhythmias with decreased myocardial contractility. There is a greater vagal control than sympathetic control, which is known to change with age. Thus, CVDs have variations among men and women, which in turn could have an effect on survival (Table 1).

BOX 1 Risk factors

Risk factors in men	Risk factors in women
• Age • Hypertension • Total cholesterol • Low density lipoprotein cholesterol	• Systolic arterial hypertension • Smoking • Diabetes • Triglyceride • High density lipoprotein cholesterol

Table 1: Gender differences in cardiovascular syndromes

Syndrome	Specific features
Myocardial infarction	Lag of 15 years in women than men with major risk factors in women being diabetes and hypertension
Hypertension	Prevalence increases steeply after menopause
Heart failure	Prevalence lower in women than men with important risk factors being diabetes and hypertension
Sudden death	More common in men

In women, CVDs have a more morbid course when it occurs at a relatively earlier age. Women with lower physical activity have a five times higher risk of mortality.

MENOPAUSE

Estrogens by acting through genomic and nongenomic mechanisms have protective effects against atherosclerosis, thus placing women at a lower risk. With menopause and decreasing estrogen, endothelial dysfunction, imbalance in autonomic activity with increased adrenergic tone, increase in visceral adiposity, and the resulting systemic inflammation leads to systemic hypertension, impaired glucose tolerance, abnormal lipid profile, and insulin resistance. Thus, menopause by itself is an independent contributor of CVD.

DYSLIPIDEMIA

Low density lipoprotein: Low estrogen downregulates the low density lipoprotein (LDL) receptors in the liver and causes decreased clearance of LDL cholesterol. Thus, between 40 and 60 years of age, there is an average increase in LDL of 0.05 mmol/L/year which does not plateau in women over 50 years of age (it plateaus in men).

High density lipoprotein: There is 4.7% decrease in the incidence of coronary artery disease in women with an increase in the high density lipoprotein cholesterol by 0.025 mmol/L as demonstrated by Framingham Heart Study and Lipid Research Clinics Prevalence Mortality Follow-up study by Gordon et al.

Triglycerides: The high triglyceride accounts for a 37% increased risk in women of CVDs.

BLOOD PRESSURE

In women, the faster pulse rate and lower diastolic blood pressure is attributed to shorter stature and shorter arterial tree. Left ventricular hypertrophy and symptomatic heart failure with preserved ejection fraction are more common in women with hypertension compared to men. There is a steep age related stiffening of the arterial wall with reduced plasma renin and angiotensin converting enzyme activity and increased salt sensitivity after menopause/ovariectomy.

CORONARY HEART DISEASE

Epidemiology

Coronary heart disease (CHD) contributed to 17% of total deaths and 26% of adult deaths in 2001-2003, which increased to 23 and 32%, respectively, in 2010-2013 as reported by the Registrar General of India. The CHD prevalence has increased from 1 to 9-10% in urban population and less than 1 to 4-6% in rural population in India over the last 60 years.

Type 2 diabetes mellitus (T2DM) and metabolic syndrome is a major risk factor accounting for 9.7 and 9.2% of CVD in men and women, respectively. Obesity in adults contributed to 3.2% in men and 6.7% in women, while high blood pressure contributed 25.9 and 24.8% in men and women, respectively.

Presentation

Women report a greater proportion of unrecognized myocardial infarction, with ischemia being silent. Atypical chest pain, complaints of abdominal pain, dyspnea, nausea, and unexplained fatigue are other common presentations in women. Other existing comorbidities can mask heart attack symptoms in women as opposed to men.

Testing

In women, exercise stress testing may be less accurate with false positivity being high in young women who have a low likelihood of CHD. In contrast, single-vessel CHD, which is more common in women than in men, might not be identified by a routine exercise stress test.

Acute Coronary Syndrome

Among the 12,000 patients who were included in the Global Use of Strategies to Open Occluded Coronary Arteries (GUSTO)-II acute coronary syndrome (ACS) study, older women with ACS presentation had a higher prevalence of risk factors such as hypertension, diabetes, and hypercholesterolemia. There was a higher prevalence of microvascular endothelial dysfunction or nonstenotic atherosclerosis among women with unstable angina or non-ST-elevation myocardial infarction who accounted for a larger proportion and they did not have significant large vessels CHD. Euro Heart Survey of ACS showed that women less than 65 years are more prone than men to develop unstable angina with less likelihood of developing ST-elevation myocardial infarction compared to women more than 65 years who were more prone to have heart failure at presentation.

HEART FAILURE

Heart failure with preserved left ventricular function is more symptomatic with more number of hospitalizations in women.

ATRIAL FIBRILLATION

Atrial fibrillation contributing to stoke with high values of congestive heart failure, hypertension, age more than or equal to 75 years, diabetes mellitus, stroke (double weight) (CHADS2) score, is more frequent in women.

DIABETES MELLITUS

Androgens increase and estrogens decrease the plasma levels of endothelin-1 expression. There is exaggerated endothelin mediated vasoconstriction in women with diabetes. The development of diabetes nullates the protective effect of estrogen. In addition, the antiproliferative effects of estrogen on vascular smooth muscle cells is inhibited by hyperglycemia which causes simultaneous activation of estrogen receptor-α and estrogen receptor-β resulting in a proinflammatory environment which further accelerates atherosclerosis. There are decreased protective effects of estrogen on body fat distribution and insulin action due to oxidative stress induced by diabetes. There is increased clot formation due to higher prothrombotic fibrin profile, denser fibrin clots, and prolonged fibrinolysis. In severe coronary artery stenosis with chronic total occlusion, there is poor collateral vessel development with female sex and T2DM being independent risk factors. Among diabetics, there is a two- to fourfold risk of developing CVD which represents 65–75% of all deaths with a three to sevenfold increased risk in women as compared to two- to threefold in men.

A significant gender difference in the cardiovascular risk profile is noted, with obesity and glycosylated hemoglobin (HbA1c) levels being higher in women as opposed to smoking and alcohol consumption that were lower but more in women. When control was taken into account, the composite control of CVD risk factors (i.e., HbA1c, blood pressure, and LDL cholesterol levels) was significantly lower in women with T2DM compared with men as reported by Joni et al in South Carolina, United States.

The future risk of CVD can be prevented by a gender-based approach in diabetics which includes innovative means of counseling for behavioral change which includes aggressive management of glycemic control and comorbidities such as dyslipidemia and hypertension.

OBESITY AND CARDIOVASCULAR DISEASE

Women have more overall body fat with more subcutaneous and less intra-abdominal fat due to the effect of estrogen, which increases fat deposition in contrast to testosterone, which inhibits fat deposition. In women, leptin and adiponectin levels are higher than in men with hyperleptinemia, which is an unphysiological state in men but not in women. This is associated with a higher risk of diabetes, hypertension, and CVD. Thus, among women with CHD, metabolic syndrome was more prevalent than in men with CHD.

CONCLUSION

The trend of CVD is on the rise in women, being the leading cause of mortality. Though many aspects of the disease are similar, there are many studies to support sex and gender dimorphisms in prevalence, presenting symptoms, management, and outcomes of CVD in women and men. More studies are needed to draw definitive conclusions as to why they are present. This understanding would lead to better management protocols.

SUGGESTED READINGS

1. Srinath Reddy K, Shah B, Varghese C, Ramadoss A. Responding to the threat of chronic diseases in India. Lancet. 2005;366:1744-9.
2. Leonarda G, Gabriella L. Gender differences in cardiovascular disease. J Integr Cardiol. 2015;1(1):20-2.
3. Joshi P, Islam S, Pais P, Reddy S, Dorairaj P, Kazmi K, et al. Risk factors for early myocardial infarction in South Asians compared with individuals in other countries. JAMA. 2007;297:286-94.
4. Xavier D, Pais P, Devereaux PJ, Xie C, Prabhakaran D, Reddy KS, et al; CREATE registry investigators. Treatment and outcomesof acute coronary syndromes in India (CREATE): a prospective analysis of registry data. Lancet. 2008;371:1435-42.
5. Harikrishnan S, Leeder S, Huffman M, et al. A Race Against Time: The Challenge of Cardiovascular Disease in Developing Economies. 2nd ed. New Delhi: New Delhi Centre for Chronic Disease Control; 2014.
6. Pednekar MS, Gupta R, Gupta PC. Illiteracy, low educational status, and cardio-vascular mortality in India. BMC Public Health. 2011;11:567.
7. Soman CR1, Kutty VR, Safraj S, Vijayakumar K, Rajamohanan K, Ajayan K; PROLIFE Study Group. All-cause mortality and cardiovascular mortality in Kerala state of India: Results from a 5-year follow-up of 161,942 rural community dwelling adults. Asia Pac J Public Health. 2011;23:896-903.
8. Gupta R, Joshi P, Mohan V, Reddy KS, Yusuf S. Epidemiology and causation of coronary heart disease and stroke in India. Heart. 2008;94:16-26.

9. Vaccarino V, Badimon L, Corti R, de Wit C, Dorobantu M, Hall A, et al. Ischaemic heart disease in women: are there sexdifferences in pathophysiology and risk factors? European Society of Cardiology. Cardiovasc Res. 2011;90(1):9-17.
10. Moodithaya S, Avadhany ST. Gender differences in age-related changes in cardiac autonomic nervous function. J Aging Res. 2012:679345.
11. Gupta R, Mohan I, Narula J. Trends in Coronary Heart Disease Epidemiology in India. Ann Glob Health. 2016;82(2):307-15.
12. Alexandra KW, Jürgen H, Giovanni P. Sex and gender differences in risk, pathophysiology and complications of type 2 diabetes mellitus. Endocr Rev. 2016; 37(3):278-316.
13. Satyavani K, Archana S, Kumar AM, Achanta S, Viswanathan V. Sex Differences in Cardiovascular Risk Factors among People with Diabetes in South India. J Assoc Physicians India. 2015;63(12):20-24.
14. Strom Williams JL, Lynch CP, Winchester R, Thomas L, Keith B, Egede LE. Gender differences in composite control of cardiovascular risk factors among patients with type 2 diabetes. Diabetes Technol Ther. 2014;16:421-7.
15. Cameron AJ, Magliano DJ, Söderberg S. A systematic review of the impact of including both waist and hip circumference in risk models for cardiovascular diseases, diabetes and mortality. Obes Rev. 2013;14(1):86-94.
16. Lilja M, Rolandsson O, Norberg M, Söderberg S. The impact of leptin and adiponectin on incident type 2 diabetes is modified by sex and insulin resistance. Metab Syndr Relat Disord. 2012;10(2):143-51.
17. Rider OJ, Lewandowski A, Nethononda R, Petersen SE, Francis JM, Pitcher A, et al. Gender specific differences in left ventricular remodelling in obesity: insights from cardiovascular magnetic resonance imaging. Eur Heart J. 2013;34(4):292-9.
18. Xin S, Adam GT, Björn Z, Yudkin JS, Söderberg S, Laatikainen T, et al. Obesity attenuates gender differences in cardiovascular mortality. Cardiovasc Diabetol. 2014;13:144.
19. Manjunath CN, Srinivas P, Ravindranath KS, Dhanalakshmi C. Incidence and patterns of valvular heart disease in a tertiary care high-volume cardiac center: A single center experience. Indian Heart J. 2014;66:320-6.
20. Yusuf, S. Hawken S, Ounpuu S, Dans T, Avezum A, Lanas F, et al. Effect of potentially modifiable riskfactors associated with myocardial infarction in 52countries (the INTERHEART study): case-control study. Lancet. 2004;36:937-52.

12

CHAPTER

Diabetic Nephropathy

Vijay Viswanathan, Anitha Rani

INTRODUCTION

Globally, among women, diabetes is ninth leading cause of death, and second highest in South Asian mortality in women with diabetes. There is remarkable gender discrimination in assessing the healthcare services and support for diabetes which lead to increased rate of mortality and morbidity in diabetic women. The long-term burden of diabetes falls inexplicably on women and they experience higher mortality and morbidity due to complications of diabetes than their male counterparts.

DIABETIC NEPHROPATHY

Diabetic nephropathy is the common cause of end-stage renal disease (ESRD) and also influences cardiovascular mortality and morbidity. Nearly 60% of the adolescent girls with diabetes are more likely to develop microalbuminuria than boys. Diabetic nephropathy is diagnosed earlier in women rather than men and more than 25% of the women with diabetic nephropathy were diagnosed during pregnancy. Furthermore, women with existing diabetic nephropathy showed increased protein excretion, which is due to pregnancy related, increased glomerular filtration in early pregnancy. This may increase the chances of earlier manifestation of diabetic nephropathy; though pregnancy does not adversely affect the course of early diabetic renal disease. The Diabetes Control and Complications Trial emphasized that the intensive control of hyperglycemia effectively delays the onset and progression of the diabetic retinopathy and nephropathy, respectively. It is also evident that the degree of proteinuria, dyslipidemia, blood pressure, and insulin requirement is higher among women with poor glycemic control. Thus, women had more abnormal manifestations of type 2 diabetes mellitus (T2DM) and nephropathy than men.

GENDER DIFFERENCE

A gender difference has been well documented in the field of nephrology. Women live longer compared to men. Proteinuria is a well known risk factor for cardiovascular disease (CVD) and mortality. Declining estimated glomerular filtration rate (eGFR) increases the rate of mortality among patients with ESRD. Estimated glomerular filtration rate is recognized and widely accepted as a major risk factor for CVD. Increased incidence of malignancy and infection may be due to chronic kidney disease (CKD). When focusing the gender difference in CKD, we should note that the eGFR is based on the patient's gender, among other variables. Modification of diet in renal disease and CKD epidemiology collaboration equations are commonly used to access the eGFR, both of these equations use gender as a variable. These are based on the assumption of the creatinine value that males have higher levels of kidney function than females, due to the fact that high muscle mass increases the generation of creatinine in males. There is a paucity of studies which uses the gold standard measurement for GFR glomerular filtration rate (GFR), and the findings based gender difference in CKD is often biased as these equations are gender dependent. Recent annual report of the United States Renal Data System showed that the prevalence of chronic renal failure was higher in females (15.1%) than males (12.1%). One should also note that in health population, as age increases, there will be a natural decline of GFR.

In general, female are protected against ESRD, thus the cumulative ESRD incidence is low during the reproductive ages and increases 10 years later in females when compare to males. Epidemiological cross-sectional data point to a higher risk of proteinuria and renal disease in women than men, among T2DM subjects. Earlier studies highlighted that the T2DM women are affected disproportionately. In general, glycemic control was poor among T2DM women and are less likely to reach target glycosylated hemoglobin.

GENDER AND DISEASE PROGRESSION

The progression of diabetic nephropathy is faster in men and often undergoes dialysis. Perhaps the mortality risk is higher among women with diabetic nephropathy than diabetic men during chronic dialysis treatment. An observational study showed that gender difference plays a major role in the progression of target organ damage among patients with insulin resistance and highlighted that the vascular and renal damage is increased in women especially women with diabetes than men. Further mortality is increased in women with diabetes and ESRD, specifically in first 4 years after dialysis. Increased inflammation and oxidative stress were observed more in diabetic women with ESRD than men, further modifiable gender difference, access, and modality of treatment were identified as risk factors for increased mortality in women with diabetes. Albuminuria is considered as a strong risk factor for CVD among T2DM males rather than female. These variations may be due to gender difference in factors like hypertension. Obesity also plays a major role in developing CKD among women than men. In addition, genetic factors also may influence the risk of developing nephropathy in women and men.

MORTALITY

All cause mortality was higher in women with diabetes. In men with T2DM, the mortality rate due to CVD has declined compared with nondiabetic men but still threefold increase due to diabetes. The risk of CVD decreased among nondiabetic women, however it did not declined in T2DM women and remains fourfold higher. The exact reason behind this gender difference remains unclear and the diabetes guideline for the treatment of diabetes also does not differentiate between genders. Literature showed that the risk of mortality is reduced more in women patients with CKD than men. The most common cause of mortality among CKD patients were CVD, infections and cancer. Recent study assessed the gender influence on CKD incidence, among patients with diabetes, and the findings highlighted that incidence of CKD is significantly increased in women rather than men.

The gender influence in diabetic nephropathy is much more debatable. Many studies showed that males are in high risk for diabetic kidney disease, whereas other studies highlighted that the females are at high risk in developing kidney disease. However, a recent study was designed to assess the gender influence on the incidence of CKD and the finding emphasized that the women with diabetes has a higher incidence of CKD. Further, women with diabetes showed high incidence of microalbuminuria. This might be due to the imbalance in hormones associated with diabetes. Preclinical evidences suggested the estrogen protects against nephropathy, as it inhibits the renin-angiotensin-aldosterone system, perhaps testosterone upregulates this system.

CONCLUSION

Apart from the conflicting data on the gender influence on diabetic nephropathy, some conclusions can be made. The prevalence of diabetic nephropathy tends to be higher in women with diabetes, but the severity of the disease is more in men. To conclude, current evidences suggested the influence of gender on diabetic nephropathy is contradictory, although it seems that the protective role of female sex on kidney is lost in diabetic kidney disease. This might be due to the association imbalance of sex hormones in diabetes. Further research is essential to understand the appropriate role of gender and its association with renal disease and its severity.

SUGGESTED READINGS

1. Carrero JJ, de Mutsert R, Axelsson J, Dekkers OM, Jager KJ, Boeschoten EW, et al. Sex differences in the impact of diabetes on mortality in chronic dialysis patients. Nephrol Dial Transplant. 2011;26(1):270-6.
2. Cohen E, Fraser A, Goldberg E, Milo G, Garty M, Krause I. Association between the body mass index and chronic kidney disease in men and women. A population-based study from Israel. Nephrol Dial Transplant. 2013;28(Suppl 4):iv130-5.
3. DCCT Research Group. Effect of intensive diabetes treatment on the development and progression of long-term complications in adolescents with insulin-dependent diabetes mellitus: Diabetes Control and Complications Trial. J Pediatr. 1994;125:177-88.
4. Gómez-Marcos MÁ, Recio-Rodríguez JI, Gómez-Sánchez L, Agudo-Conde C, Rodríguez-Sanchez E, Maderuelo-Fernandez J, et al. Gender differences in the progression of target organ damage in patients with increased insulin resistance: the LOD-DIABETES study. Cardiovasc Diabetol. 2015;14:132.
5. Hecking M, Bieber BA, Ethier J, Kautzky-Willer A, Sunder-Plassmann G, Säemann MD, et al. Sex-specific differences in hemodialysis prevalence and practices and the male-to-female mortality rate: the Dialysis Outcomes and Practice Patterns Study (DOPPS). PLoS Med. 2014;11(10):e1001750.
6. Komura H, Nomura I, Kitamura K, Kuwasako K, Kato J. Gender difference in relationship between body mass index and development of chronic kidney disease. BMC Res Notes. 2013;6(1):463.
7. Maric C. Sex, diabetes and the kidney. Am J Physiol Renal Physiol. 2009;296(4):F680-8.
8. Pounds LL, Teodorescu VJ. Chronic kidney disease and dialysis access in women. J Vasc Surg. 2013;57(4 Suppl):49-53S.
9. Roche MM, Wang PP. Sex differences in all-cause and cardiovascular mortality, hospitalization for individuals with and without diabetes, and patients with diabetes diagnosed early and late. Diabetes Care. 2013;36(9):2582-90.
10. Szalat A, Raz I. Gender-specific care of diabetes mellitus: particular considerations in the management of diabetic women. Diabetes Obes Metab. 2008;10(12):1135-56.
11. United States Renal Data System. (2015). 2015 USRDS annual data report: Epidemiology of kidney disease in the United States. National Institutes of Health, National Institute of Diabetes and Digestive and Kidney Diseases. [online] Available from: http://www.usrds.org/adr.aspx. [Accessed April, 2017].
12. Zoppini G, Targher G, Chonchol M, Perrone F, Lippi G, Muggeo M. Higher HDL cholesterol levels are associated with a lower incidence of chronic kidney disease in patients with type 2 diabetes. Nutr Metab Cardiovasc Dis. 2009;19(8):580-6.

13

CHAPTER

Diabetic Neuropathy

Sweta Singla, Deepak Khandelwal

INTRODUCTION

Diabetes has gained pandemic proportions. The recent estimates suggest approximately 422 million people (aged 20–79 years) worldwide to be suffering from diabetes mellitus, with global prevalence being 8.8%. By 2040, these figures are projected to be 642 million, with a prevalence of 10.4%. Genderwise, male diabetic population (215.2 million) is slightly higher than female diabetic population (199.5 million). Prevalence is similar in both genders till 60 years of age after which women have higher prevalence. With women having a longer lifespan, the number of diabetic women is rising with recent increase in life expectancy. Gender disparities do exist in terms of diabetes care, access to healthcare and support especially in developing countries like India. World Health Organization (WHO) reports that 55% of deaths related to diabetes occurs in women.

For India, WHO estimates diabetes prevalence to be more in men (7.9%) as compared to women (7.5%), despite more Indian women being overweight (23.9% vs. 19% in males), obese (6.5% in women vs. 3.1% in men), and more prone to physical inactivity (15.1% vs. 9.2% in men). However, after age standardization, there is no gender difference in these figures.

Diabetic neuropathy (DN) is one of the most common and disabling complications of diabetes. The estimates of DN prevalence vary widely from 9.6 to 78% in different populations. Earlier landmark trials have shown high prevalence of DN [66% in Rochester DN Study and 39% in Diabetes Control and Complications Trial (DCCT)]. Prevalence in Indian studies has been found to be varying from 9.1 to 29.2%. Such wide differences are due to use of different methodology and definitions of neuropathy used in different studies. As compared to European populations, Indians have lower prevalence of both large and small fiber neuropathy but 50% higher chances of developing painful neuropathy.

GENDER DIFFERENCES IN DIABETIC NEUROPATHY

Data on gender differences in prevalence of DN has been scarce and is inconsistent. Most of the earlier studies were not planned to study gender-based differences. Gender differences were noticed in DCCT where electrophysiological abnormalities or nerve conduction study abnormalities were more consistently correlated with clinical neuropathy in males as compared to females.

A recent Indian study found similar prevalence of DN in both genders (29.3% in women vs. 29.1% in men). Similar studies from Pakistan by Javed et al. and Srilanka by Katulanda et al. did not find any gender difference in prevalence of diabetic peripheral neuropathy. However, few retrospective studies (Aaberg et al. and Kamenov et al.) have shown higher prevalence and earlier onset of DN in men. Postulated reasons for same are differences in lifestyle, with more hazardous lifestyle in men including stressful jobs, higher smoking habits, higher frequency of alcohol and drugs use, and lower compliance with treatment.

PHYSIOLOGICAL AND PATHOLOGICAL DIFFERENCES IN MALES AND FEMALES

Important physiological and pathophysiological sex differences exist in terms of anthropometric, biochemical, metabolic, and endocrine parameters. These factors interplay an important role in the clinical manifestations of diabetes and its complications. Female child is born lighter and is proposed to be genetically more prone to be resistant to trophic effects of the insulin. Diabetic women are more obese than diabetic men in most studies and show a stronger association between increase of body mass index and diabetes risk. Sex differences in body composition and fat deposition clearly contribute to sex-dimorphic diabetes risk. Women have higher activity of brown adipose tissue as compared to males. The balanced proportion between estrogen and androgen plays an important role in maintenance of energy metabolism, body composition, and sexual function.

SOCIOECONOMIC GENDER DIFFERENCES AND ITS IMPLICATION ON DIABETES AND ITS COMPLICATIONS

In India, women have a very different social environment and stature as compared to men, with disparities more prominent in rural as compared to urban regions. Women's health is usually put on the back-burner not only by her family but the women themselves. Females usually under-report symptoms, are less likely to adhere to clinic visits, less likely to care for dietary restrictions, or to take nutritious food. Men are more likely to consume both tobacco and alcohol while obesity and low intake of fruit and vegetables are more common in women.

Weaver and Hadley (2011) published an extensive list of stress reported by women with diabetes and discussed how these stressor result from and contribute to social roles and mental distress. Sridhar and Madhu (2002) found that men more commonly relied on their spouses to manage their diets and are less likely to seek their support with regard to emotional states or medication adherence. Men are more likely to adjust and integrate diabetes into their lives than their female counterparts, and hence, have better quality of life (QoL).

The gender differences gain more importance in lower socioeconomic strata, where males are the bread winners and women are dependent on them as per the cultural norms. Diabetes being a chronic illness has a monthly financial burden on a household. Because of this chronic expense, diabetic women experience stress of being a burden on the monthly budget. Apart from financial stress, females both from low and middle-income women report concerns regarding interpersonal abuse, loneliness, burden of alcoholic spouse, and co-occurring depression. These factors also lead to poor management of diabetes in female diabetics.

PATHOPHYSIOLOGICAL FACTORS THAT LEAD TO DIABETES NEUROPATHY AND HOW THEY ARE DIFFERENT IN MALES VERSUS FEMALES

The pathogenesis of DN is multifactorial. The various pathogenic factors are often interrelated and together contribute to the development and progression of neuropathy. Major mechanisms involved in the pathogenesis of DN are hyperglycemia, local nerve ischemia, neurotrophic factors deficiencies, and immune dysregulation. Other mechanisms contributing are increased activity of protein kinase C and decreased synthesis of γ-linolenic acid. Long-term metformin use may be an iatrogenic cause of neuropathy.

There is no literature to support that any of these mechanisms has any gender difference to predispose specific gender to higher risk of neuropathy.

Regarding risk factors for DN, in DCCT, apart from male sex, taller subjects, longer duration of diabetes, increasing age, presence of retinopathy, and lower stimulated C-peptide levels were found to be risk factors significantly associated with neuropathy development. Broadly, the distribution of the various types of DN varies according to the population studied and the methodology used. In Rochester Diabetes Neuropathy study, out of the 66% of the total study subjects, who were found to have DN, the frequencies of individual types were as follows—polyneuropathy, 54%; carpal tunnel syndrome, asymptomatic, 22%, and symptomatic, 11%; visceral autonomic neuropathy, 7%; and other varieties, 3%. No significant gender differences have been reported apart from entrapment neuropathy which is more prevalent in women. Females with the smaller wrist size and frequent wrist movements during their domestic chores are predisposed to entrapment neuropathy even in nondiabetic population.

VULVODYNIA: AN UNRECOGNIZED DIABETIC NEUROPATHIC SYNDROME

Recently interest has been generated by the description of new type of neuropathy in diabetic women that is characterized as vulvar pain. Kalra et al. in their review described unexplained vulvar pain or vulvodynia as a manifestation of painful sensory DN, which is a common source of morbidity in women. Vulvodynia may be unilateral or bilateral in its distribution. It may present as an isolated symptom or as a part of constellation of other neuropathic abnormalities. Vulvodynia may be due to other illnesses like herpetic neuralgia and female sexual dysfunction, which are also otherwise more common in diabetics.

DIABETIC NEUROPATHY AND QUALITY OF LIFE AND ITS GENDER IMPLICATIONS

Diabetic neuropathy compromises the QoL by multiple mechanisms including pain associated with painful DN, loss of autonomic homeostasis, and by increasing the rate of further complication like foot ulcerations and risk of amputation. Almost 40–50% of patients with DN have significant painful neuropathic symptoms, which is an important cause of morbidity in these patients.

Females are more disabled with DN and suffer greater deterioration in QoL index. In one of the largest study on DN in Romania on diabetic patients from 51 cities, gender differences in QoL perception were evaluated in patients with self-reported diabetes with and without neuropathy. Females consistently reported higher burden on QoL even though males had higher frequency of DN complications, like foot ulcers, gangrene, and amputations.

THERAPEUTICS STRATEGIES: GENDER IMPLICATIONS

Diabetes Management

The most important step in the management of any DN is strict glycemic control. Landmark clinical trials like DCCT and United Kingdom Prospective Diabetes Study (UKPDS) have shown that meticulous glycemic control not only decreases the risk of developing neuropathy but also slows the progression in established neuropathy. Management of hyperglycemia in patients with neuropathy is generally on same lines as patients without neuropathy. As patients with neuropathy may have concomitant nephropathy, they may require appropriate dose adjustment of various oral hypoglycemics (OHA). Also some OHA may be contraindicated depending on renal function. Many patients with severe hyperglycemia and painful DN benefit with short-term insulin therapy, although insulin is not mandatory in all cases with neuropathy. On the other hand, sudden control of hyperglycemic state sometimes may worsen neuropathic symptoms transiently, called as insulin neuritis. Fluctuations in blood glucose need to be avoided and stable control of glycemia is desired. Gender differences in terms of side effect profile may be seen with some OHA; like genital fungal infections with the use of sodium-glucose cotransporter (SGLT)-2 inhibitors occur significantly more often in females.

Neuropathy Management

Most important factor in the management of DN is good glycemic control as discussed in previous section. Other comorbidities like hypovitaminosis B12, smoking, alcoholism, and dyslipidemia need to addressed, if patient has any of these associated comorbidities. Other reversible/secondary causes of neuropathy like autoimmune/infectious and parainfectious causes need to be excluded before labeling a diagnosis of DN. As the management strategies are primarily palliative rather than curative, prevention of the clinical neuropathy is important. Therapeutic agents like aldose reductase inhibitor, α-lipoic acid, and angiotensin converting enzyme inhibitors have been tried but have not shown consistent benefits in clinical studies.

In painful diabetic neuropathic pain (DNP), symptomatic management consists of pain relief. Tricyclic antidepressants, serotonin and norepinephrine reuptake inhibitors like venlafaxine and duloxetine, antiepileptic drugs like gabapentin and pregabalin are the commonly used pharmaceutical agents for painful DNP. In resistant cases, narcotics like opioids or benzodiazepines may be tried. Other therapeutic modalities that are effective include local lidocaine, capsaicin cream, acupuncture, and transcutaneous electric nerve stimulation. As far as gender difference is concerned, the above modalities work equally well in males and females.

CONCLUSION

Well-planned studies regarding gender differences for DN are scarce at present. There exist some differences in prevalence, types, and manifestations of DN in females as compared to males. Therapeutic strategies may need to be modified as per gender. Future well-planned studies are required in this area to answer many questions. With the newly described presentations of neuropathy like vulvodynia, a lot many aspects of neuropathy appear unexplored.

SUGGESTED READINGS

1. Aaberg ML, Burch DM, Hud ZR, et al. Gender differences in the onset of diabetic neuropathy. J Diabetes Complications. 2008;22(2):83-7.
2. Bajaj S, Jawad F, Islam N, et al. South Asian women with diabetes: Psychosocial challenges and management: Consensus statement. Indian J Endocr Metab. 2013;17:548-62.
3. Deli G, Bosnyak E, Pusch G, et al. Diabetic Neuropathies: Diagnosis and Management. Neuroendocrinology. 2013;98:267-80.
4. Athar J, Ahmad F, Mohsin Z, et al. Gender based differences in diabetic peripheral neuropathy. Pakistan J Neurol Sci. 2014;9(4):20-4.
5. Kalra B, Kalra S, Bajaj S. Vulvodynia: An unrecognized diabetic neuropathic syndrome. Indian J Endocr Metab. 2013;17:787-9.
6. Kamenov ZA, Parapunova RA, Georgieva RT. Earlier development of diabetic neuropathy in men than in women with type 2 diabetes mellitus. Gend Med. 2010;7:600-5.
7. Kautzky-Willer A, Harreiter J, Pacini G. Sex and Gender Differences in Risk, Pathophysiology and Complications of Type 2 Diabetes Mellitus. Endocr Rev. 2016;37(3):278-316.
8. Mendenhall E, Shivashankar R, Tandon N, et al. Stress and Diabetes in Socioeconomic Context: A Qualitative Study of Urban Indians. Soc sci med. 2012;75(12):2522-9.
9. Sridhar G, Madhu K, Veena S, et al. Living with diabetes: Indian experience. Diabetes Metabol Syndrome. 2007;1:181-7.
10. Sridhar G, Madhu K. Psychosocial and cultural issues in diabetes mellitus. Curr Sci. 2002;83:

14

CHAPTER

Infections

Jayanta K Panda, Madhusmita Patnaik

INTRODUCTION

Diabetes mellitus is a clinical syndrome characterized by deficiency of insulin secretion or its action. It is one of the greatest emerging dangers to human healthcare in the 21st century. It is calculated that there will be 380 million people suffering from diabetes in 2025.

In addition to the serious complications of the disease, it has been associated with decreased effects of T cells, neutrophil function, and disorders of humoral immunity. Thus, diabetes mellitus increases the susceptibility to infections and it may stimulate diabetes mellitus complications such as ketoacidosis and hypoglycemia. The belief of the association between diabetes mellitus and increased susceptibility to infection is not supported by strong evidence. Although many specific infections are more common in diabetic patients and some occur almost exclusively in diabetics. Few infections occur with increased severity and are associated with an increased risk of complications in diabetics. Infections in a diabetic woman at India are various. Some infections are more common in diabetic woman than men. The common infections associated with diabetic women in our country are asymptomatic bacteriuria, urinary tract infection, emphysematous pyelonephritis, emphysematous cystitis, vulvovaginitis, and hepatitis-C infection. Such type of infections are reviewed in this chapter. The aim of this article is to assess the recent facts on the infections associated with the diabetics and to describe the common infections associated with diabetic women of India.

MATERIALS AND METHODS

All published articles were searched from 1998 and 2017, using different keywords like "diabetes mellitus and infection," "infections of diabetic

BOX 1 Infections commonly associated with diabetes mellitus

Respiratory infections
- *Streptococcus pneumoniae*
- Influenza
- H1N1
- Tuberculosis

Urinary tract infections
- Asymptomatic bacteriuria
- Fungal cystitis
- Emphysematous cystitis
- Perinephric abscess

Gastrointestinal and liver infections
- Helicobacter pylori infection
- Oral and esophageal candidiasis
- Emphysematous cholecystitis
- Hepatitis C
- Hepatitis B
- *Enteroviruses*

Skin and soft tissue infections
- Foot infection
- Necrotizing fasciitis
- Fournier's gangrene

Head and neck infections
- Invasive external otitis
- Rhinocerebral mucormycosis

Other infections
- Human immunodeficiency

women," "infection of Indian diabetic women." Search for papers included both original articles and review articles. They were included on the presence of relevant titles and abstracts. The articles without abstract and relevant titles to the basis of this review were excluded.

THE SPECTRUM OF INFECTIOUS DISEASES OCCURRING IN PATIENTS WITH DIABETES (BOX 1)

Common infections in diabetic patients are—respiratory tract infection mostly community acquired pneumonia. Urinary tract infection, mostly acute bacterial cystitis, acute pyelonephritis, emphysematous pyelonephritis, perinephric abscess, and fungal cystitis. Skin and soft tissue infection, mostly necrotizing fasciitis. Abdominal infection mostly emphysematous cholecystitis. Others are invasive otitis external, rhinocerebral mucormycosis.

Most of the controlled studies have proved that infection incidence rate is higher in diabetic women than in nondiabetic women.

DIABETES MELLITUS AND INFECTION: PATHOPHYSIOLOGY (FLOWCHART 1)

Chronic hyperglycemia along with presence of glycemic complications result in impairment of host defense mechanisms and facilitates the growth of various aerobic and anaerobic microorganisms, thereby causing infections in diabetes patients. The most common pathological mechanisms

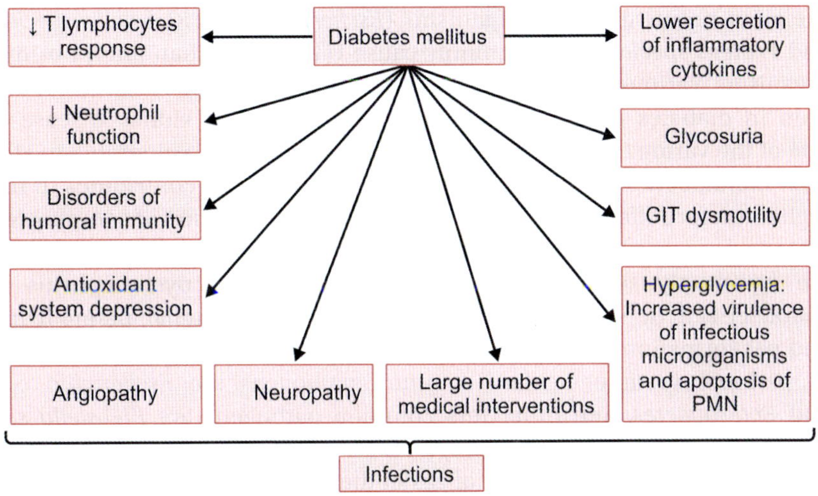

GIT, gastrointestinal tract; PMN, polymorphonuclear leukocyte.

FLOWCHART 1: Diabetes mellitus and infection: Pathophysiology

for infections are high glucose level increases the virulence of organisms; decreased production of interleukins; reduced chemotaxis, adherence and phagocytic activity; immobilization of polymorphonuclear leukocytes; glycosuria; urinary and gastrointestinal dysmotility, etc.

URINARY TRACT INFECTION

Women suffering from diabetes mellitus have high risk of asymptomatic bacteriuria, urinary tract infection (UTI), emphysematous pyelonephritis, and emphysematous cystitis. Urinary tract infections in diabetes mellitus cause most common bacterial infection among women resulting high incidence of hospitalization. More susceptible persons for UTIs in general are the elderly, spinal cord injury patients on catheters, people with multiple sclerosis, human immunodeficiency virus infected individuals, as well as diabetes mellitus patients. Female diabetic patients have higher prevalence of lower UTI than male type 2 diabetes mellitus (T2DM) patient. Different epidemiological studies revealed the evidence of UTI is more common in diabetic women than nondiabetic women. The number of microorganisms situated in the vagina are responsible for high level of infection in the urinary tract of diabetic women. Recent studies (Jenifer et al.) shows asymptomatic bacteriuria was more common with diabetic women (26%) than nondiabetic women (6%). Special care is needed for the management of bacterial UTIs as the diabetic women have high risk of suffering from UTIs. Various risk factors are associated with UTIs such as old age, sexual intercourse, long duration of diabetes, poor glycemic control, and complications of diabetes. Bacteriological studies mostly revealed the gram negative enteric organisms (*Escherichia coli, Klebsiella species,* and *Proteus species*) are commonly cause UTIs rather than gram positive organisms. Various long-term effects on the genitourinary system has been seen in diabetes mellitus. The complication diabetic kidney disease is one of the various causes that help these patients more vulnerable to UTI than nondiabetics. Reduced immunity in diabetes also contributes to the higher risk for suffering UTI. Some uncommon presentation of complicated UTIs such as emphysematous pyelonephritis and emphysematous cystitis are commonly seen in diabetics. Emphysematous pyelonephritis is characterized by severe necrotizing infection of the renal parenchyma and gas formation within the collecting system, renal parenchyma, and/or perinephric tissues. Most common pathogens are *Escherichia coli* and *Enterobacter*, and other less common pathogens are *Klebsiella sp., Proteus sp., Candida sp.,* and *Streptococcus sp.* Emphysematous cystitis is characterized by the formation of gas in the bladder wall and cavity due to infection by bacteria which produce carbon dioxide. *Escherichia coli* is most common pathogen and other less common pathogens are *Enterobacter, Proteus, Klebsiella,* and *Candida*.

VULVOVAGINAL INFECTION

Symptomatic vulvovaginal candidiasis has been proven to be more common in diabetic women than nondiabetic women. Predisposing factor for vulvovaginal infection in women, especially vaginal candidiasis, are diabetes, obesity, oral contraceptives of high estrogen dose, pregnancy, drug addiction, and use of broad-spectrum antibiotics. The possible etiology of recurrent infections is the poor management of glucose level in diabetic women that reduces several aspects of humoral host defense and decreases chemotaxis, phagocytosis, immobilization of neutrophils, and killing of microbials. *Candida albicans* is found to be a predominant and the most virulent species in symptomatic group of patients followed by *Candida glabrata*, while in asymptomatic group of patients, *Candida krusei* is predominant. Most of the individuals mean age of 40–51 years with vaginal candidiasis infection are suffering from T2DM, while in type 1 diabetes mellitus (T1DM), it occurs before 30 and during pregnancy. Vaginal candidiasis infection does not cause severe symptoms always and sometimes it present with no symptoms or very mild symptoms.

HEPATITIS C VIRUS INFECTION

Among American-Indian women, T2DM is more common with hepatitis C virus (HCV) infection than those without HCV infection. Hepatitis C virus positive individuals are three times more likely to develop diabetes mellitus than the negative. This correlation is independent of age and body mass index. Therefore, T2DM is included an extrahepatic manifestation of HCV infection. It is seen that the patients with HCV infection who develop diabetes mellitus have more severe liver disease and increased fibrosis compared to nondiabetic HCV patients. A genetic predisposition of individuals to T2DM may be a possible explanation. So, HCV infection could cause: (i) a direct viral effect, mostly genotype 1 or 4 suppress the ß-cell function and/or (ii) a liver damage lead to abnormal glucose metabolism and insulin resistance. Therefore, early screening of HCV infection and T2DM in HCV infected individuals should be required for all susceptible patients.

CONCLUSION

Infections in a diabetic women are more common than in diabetic men. Various epidemiological studies also revealed that infection in diabetic women are more common than in nondiabetic women in India. The main infectious diseases associated with diabetic women in India are UTI, vulvovaginitis, and diabetes mellitus in HCV infection. Various risk factors are associated with infection in diabetic women such as old age, long duration of diabetes, poor glycemic control, diabetic complications, and recurrent vaginal infection. The most common pathogenic mechanisms are high glucose level increases the virulence of organisms; decreased production of interleukins; reduced chemotaxis, adherence and phagocytic activity; immobilization of neutrophils; glycosuria; urinary and gastrointestinal dysmotility, etc. More research is needed for all types of infections and their pathogenesis occurring in diabetic women of India to reduce the morbidity and mortality.

SUGGESTED READINGS

1. Casquiro J, Casquiro J, Alves C. Infections in patients with diabetes mellitus: A review of pathogenesis. Indian J Endocrinol Metab. 2012;16 Suppl 1:S27-36.
2. Eshwarappa M, Dosegowda R, Aprameya IV, et al. Clinico-microbiological profile of urinary tract infection in south India. Indian J Nephrol. 2011;21:30-6.
3. Janifer J, Geethalakshmi S, Satyavani K, et al. Prevalence of lower urinary tract infection in south Indian type 2 diabetic subjects. Indian J Nephrol. 2009;19:107-18.
4. Joshi N, Caputo GM, Weitecamp MR, et al. Infections in patient with diabetes mellitus. N Engl J Med. 1999;341(25):1906-12.
5. Reza Faraji R, Rahimi MA, Rezvanmadani F, et al. Prevalence of vaginal candidiasis infection in diabetic women. African Journal of Microbiology Research. 2012;6(11): 2773-8.
6. Shrivastav VK, Shukla D, Shrivastav A, et al. Prevalence of vaginal candidiasis in diabetic women of Madhya Pradesh, India. Int J Curr Microbiol App Sci. 2015;4(5): 834-46.
7. Wilson C. Hepatitis C infection and type 2 diabetes in American-Indian women. Diabetes Care. 2004;27(9):2116-9.

15
CHAPTER

Polycystic Ovary Syndrome

SR Aravind, Chitra Selvan

INTRODUCTION

Polycystic ovary syndrome (PCOS) is one of the most common endocrine abnormalities in women of reproductive age with a prevalence ranging from 5 to 11%. While the name may disarmingly suggest that it is primarily a reproductive or gynecological disorder, it is in fact a heterogenous endocrine disorder with some serious metabolic consequences like predisposition to type 2 diabetes mellitus (T2DM) and coronary artery disease.

The pathogenesis of PCOS is at large, poorly understood but it is accepted that insulin resistance has an undeniable role to play. In this chapter, we review the definition and clinical manifestations of PCOS, its pathogenesis and the relationship with diabetes and comprehensive care.

POLYCYSTIC OVARY SYNDROME: PREVALENCE IN INDIA

The prevalence of PCOS in India has been to be similar to and in some instances higher than that reported worldwide ranging from 3.7 to 22.5%, with 9–36% prevalence in adolescents alone. Considering the rise in obesity in our population, the prevalence of PCOS is only expected to increase.

POLYCYSTIC OVARY SYNDROME: DEFINITION AND CLINICAL MANIFESTATIONS

The most common clinical features of PCOS are irregular cycles, acne, hirsutism, and infertility. Thus, patients with PCOS present to various specialties like dermatology, gynecology, infertility specialists, physicians, and endocrinologists, and most times, this means they miss out on a holistic comprehensive long-term care.

The diagnostic criteria most commonly followed is the Rotterdam criteria by The European Society of Human Reproduction and Embryology/ American Society for Reproductive Medicine (ESHRE/ASRM). The diagnosis of PCOS is made when two of the following three conditions are met:

1. Clinical and/or biochemical hyperandrogenemia
   - Biochemical: Serum total testosterone
   - Clinical: Persistent acne, hirsutism
2. Oligo and/or anovulation
3. Polycystic ovaries on ultrasound.

Hirsutism is the excessive growth of thick, dark terminal hair in the androgen dependent areas of the body. It is one of the clinical manifestations of hyperandrogenemia. Commonly affected and assessed sites are—upper lip, chin, chest, abdomen, thighs, upper and lower back, and upper arms. The modified Ferriman-Gallaway score is used to quantify the hirsutism score. The presence of fine, thin vellous hair over the forearms or calf region is not hirsutism. Acne and temporal balding are also a clinical manifestation of hyperandrogenemia.

Biochemical hyperadrogenemia is usually assessed by measuring serum total testosterone levels, calculating free androgen levels or measuring dihydroepiandrostenedione sulfate levels.

Oligo/anovulation is defined as cycle length more than or equal to 35 days.

Polycystic ovary morphology as defined by ESHRE/ASRM consensus criteria is as at least one ovary with more than or equal to 12 follicles of 2–9 mm (between days 2–5 of cycle) or ovarian volume greater than 10 mL in the absence of a cyst or dominant follicle greater than 10 mm, established with ultrasound examination of ovaries.

The diagnosis of PCOS can only be made when conditions which can mimic PCOS have been excluded like congenital adrenal hyperplasia, Cushing's syndrome and androgen secreting tumors, hypothyroidism, and hyperprolactinemia.

PATHOGENESIS

Our understanding of the pathogenesis of PCOS is still evolving and is poorly understood as of today. Polycystic ovary syndrome is a condition with interplay of environmental factors in genetically predisposed individuals in the context of insulin resistance with dysregulated ovarian steroidogenesis leading to hyperandrogenemia, anovulation, and metabolic consequences.

Women with PCOS appear to have greater insulin resistance even after adjusting for body mass index (BMI), an observation in line with their greater visceral fat accumulation and higher waist to hip ratio compared with women without PCOS. It is important to note that insulin has effects at the level of ovary. The insulin resistance in PCOS is seen at the level of the liver, adipose tissue, and muscle whereas the ovary remains sensitive to the actions of insulin. Thus, the compensatory hyperinsulinemia in insulin-resistant states contributes to the ovarian androgen excess.

Theca cells surrounding the follicles in the ovary produce androgens in response to luteinizing hormone (LH). Androgens then diffuse from theca cells to granulosa cells, where they form substrates for estrogen formation in response to follicle stimulating hormone (FSH).

Normal thecal androgen production supports antral follicle growth and development. Androgens do so in part by upregulating granulosa cell expression of FSH receptors and then augment FSH induction of granulosa cell LH receptors, thus luteinizing granulosa cells and sensitizing them to both gonadotropins. Insulin amplifies the luteinization process. Androgen excess stimulates the excess proliferation of small antral follicles while causing follicle maturation arrest. Increased proliferation of these astral follicles further contributed to hyperandrogenemia.

While production of androgens by theca cells is sensitive to LH, the negative feedback of androgen on gonadotrophin levels in females is not very strong. This leads to increase in levels of androgens further. Antral follicle growth is accompanied by increased production of anti-Müllerian hormone, which normally acts as a gatekeeper that inhibits primordial follicles from entering the growth phase.

Insulin excess appears to fuel this process further by enabling hyper-responsiveness of the ovarian theca cells to LH.

METABOLIC EFFECTS OF POLYCYSTIC OVARY SYNDROME: THE INDIAN PERSPECTIVE

Studies on PCOS from India have reported a prevalence rate of 37.5–62.5% for obesity in patients with PCOS. Metabolic syndrome occurs in up to one-third of PCOS adolescents and nearly half of PCOS adults. Among PCOS patients, an abnormal degree of insulin resistance is reported in about one- to two-thirds. Hyperandrogenemia itself per se may be responsible for metabolic perturbations seen in PCOS. Polycystic ovary syndrome confers a substantially increased risk for T2DM and gestational diabetes from early life. About 1 in 5 women with PCOS will develop T2DM making impaired glucose tolerance (IGT) a common abnormality in this disease. The prevalence of glucose intolerance in Indian women with PCOS is reported as 16.3% (adults 19.1%, adolescents 9.7%). Furthermore, prospective longitudinal studies in young and middle-aged women with PCOS show a higher risk for developing diabetes later in life.

Interestingly, family history of diabetes increases the prevalence of T2DM in PCOS patients. However, the prevalence of diabetes in PCOS patients with no family history of diabetes was still much higher than normal women. Even though family history and obesity are major contributors in the development of diabetes in PCOS patients, diabetes can still occur in lean PCOS patients who have no family history. Thus, women with PCOS are at high risk for T2DM.

A subtype of PCOS, more commonly seen in our ethnicity, is the "lean PCOS" phenotype where the BMI is within the ethnicity-specific normal range (BMI: 18.5–22.9 kg/m^2). In a study conducted in Delhi which studied women with PCOS and compared the two groups, lean and obese PCOS, found that while their BMI were different, the central android obesity was similar in the two groups. It was also interesting to note that prevalence of hypertension were similar in the obese and nonobese group. The prevalence of impaired glucose tolerance and T2DM were greater in the obese group.

Women with PCOS are at seven times higher risk of myocardial infarction in patients with PCOS compared to healthy controls. Patients with PCOS have significantly elevated levels of circulating biomarkers of CVD, including C-reactive protein and lipoprotein A in comparison to matched controls. Other studies demonstrated a higher burden of indicators of atherosclerosis with early onset cardiovascular dysfunction, i.e., arterial stiffness, endothelial dysfunction, and coronary artery calcification.

Should Clinicians Routinely Screen for Diabetes in Women with Polycystic Ovary Syndrome?

It is recommended that all women and preferably even adolescents be screened for diabetes periodically. The oral glucose tolerance test (OGTT) (consisting of a fasting and 2-hour glucose level using a 75 g oral glucose load) is the gold standard for testing. An observational study from India reported "2-hour postglucose insulin levels" as a better indicator of insulin resistance in women with PCOS. A hemoglobin A1c (HbA1c) test may be considered if a patient is unable or unwilling to complete an OGTT. Rescreening is suggested every 3–5 years, or more frequently if clinical factors such as central adiposity, substantial weight gain, and/or symptoms of diabetes develop.

Preconception counseling should be done at every visit and patient sensitized to their higher risk for gestational diabetes and T2DM.

It is also recommended that adolescents and women with PCOS be screened for the following cardiovascular disease risk factors like hypertension and dyslipidemia in the presence of the following risk factors—family history of early cardiovascular disease, cigarette smoking, IGT/T2DM, hypertension, dyslipidemia, obstructive sleep apnea (OSA), and obesity.

POLYCYSTIC OVARY SYNDROME AND COMPREHENSIVE CARE

Women with PCOS are at increased risk for depression, OSA, and non-alcoholic fatty liver disease, hence, screening for symptoms suggestive of them is recommended. Women with PCOS are also at risk for endometrial cancer, but routine screening ultrasounds for endometrial thickness are not recommended although it may be prudent to induce uterine bleeds at periodic intervals of at least 45–60 days.

MANAGEMENT OF POLYCYSTIC OVARY SYNDROME

The management of PCOS can be dealt with under two subdivisions:

1 The sustained effort to challenge the environmental factors that contribute to the disease with an aim of improving long-term morbidities and complications
2 The specific management of the presentation relevant to the patient at that point in her life, e.g., hirsutism or acne, menstrual irregularity, or infertility.

Although there are no large randomized trials of exercise in PCOS, exercise therapy, alone or in combination with dietary intervention, improves weight loss and reduces cardiovascular risk factors and diabetes risk in the general population. Weight loss is likely beneficial for both reproductive and metabolic dysfunction in this setting.

Metformin is recommended to be used in patients with PCOS with dysglycemia who have failed lifestyle modifications. It can be used as second-line agent for women with PCOS with menstrual irregularities especially if they are intolerant to or have contraindications to hormonal contraceptives. The blanket use of metformin as a first line treatment of acne/hirsutism or for prevention of pregnancy complications, or for the treatment of obesity is discouraged.

CONCLUSION

Polycystic ovary syndrome is an endocrine disorder with myriad heterogenous presentations but with an increased risk of metabolic perturbations like gestational diabetes, T2DM, and cardiovascular disease. The periodic screening for diabetes and CV risk factors is recommended in all women and adolescents with PCOS with a special focus on prepregnancy counseling. A sustained effort to modify lifestyle to decrease long-term morbidity is to be reiterated at every encounter with the person.

SUGGESTED READINGS

1. Allahbadia GN, Merchant R. Polycystic ovary syndrome in the Indian subcontinent. Semin Reprod Med. 2008;26(1):22-34.
2. Diamanti-Kandarakis E. Polycystic ovarian syndrome: pathophysiology, molecular aspects and clinical implications. Expert Rev Mol Med. 2008;10:e3.
3. Gill H, Tiwari P, Dabadghao P. Prevalence of polycystic ovary syndrome in young women from North India: A Community-based study. Indian J Endocrinol Metab. 2012;16(Suppl 2):S389-92.
4. Joshi B, Mukherjee S, Patil A, et al. A cross-sectional study of polycystic ovarian syndrome among adolescent and young girls in Mumbai, India. Indian J Endocrinol Metab. 2014;18(3):317-24.
5. Legro RS, Arslanian SA, Ehrmann DA, et al. Diagnosis and Treatment of Polycystic Ovary Syndrome: An Endocrine Society Clinical Practice Guideline. J Clin Endocrinol Metab. 2013;98(12):4565-92.
6. Majumdar A, Singh TA. Comparison of clinical features and health manifestations in lean vs. obese Indian women with polycystic ovarian syndrome. J Hum Reprod Sci. 2009;2(1):12-7.
7. Malik S, Jain K, Talwar P, et al. Management of Polycystic Ovary Syndrome in India. Fertil Sci Res. 2014;1:23-43.
8. Nair MK, Pappachan P, Balakrishnan S, et al. Menstrual irregularity and polycystic ovarian syndrome among adolescent girls—a 2-year follow-up study. Indian J Pediatr. 2012;79 (Suppl 1):S69-S73.
9. Nidhi R, Padmalatha V, Nagarathna R, et al. Prevalence of polycystic ovarian syndrome in Indian adolescents. J Pediatr Adolesc Gynecol. 2011;24:223-7.
10. Rosenfield RL, Ehrmann DA. The Pathogenesis of Polycystic Ovary Syndrome (PCOS): The Hypothesis of PCOS as Functional Ovarian Hyperandrogenism Revisited. Endocr Rev. 2016;37(5):467-520.
11. Rotterdam ESHRE/ASRM-Sponsored PCOS Consensus Workshop Group. Revised 2003 consensus on diagnostic criteria and long-term health risks related to polycystic ovary syndrome. Fertil Steril. 2004;81(1):19-25.

16

CHAPTER

Bone Health

Ranabir Salam, Manash P Baruah

INTRODUCTION

Diabetes mellitus can affect bone health. Radiological findings of retarded bone development and bone atrophy in children with type 1 diabetes mellitus (T1DM) were reported around 90 years back. In 1952, the association between osteoporosis and diabetes was described in a case report.

In the Study of Women's Health Across the Nation (SWAN), women who had diabetes had significantly higher bone mineral density (BMD) at hip and lumbar spine. Age adjusted incident fractures were twofold higher in such women compared to nondiabetic population. In The Blue Mountains Eye Study after 2 years of follow-up, diabetes was significantly associated with increased risk of fractures.

BONE MINERAL DENSITY STUDIES IN TYPE 1 DIABETES MELLITUS

Various studies have reported conflicting reports on BMD at different sites. Some studies reporting significantly lower values among T1DM and some no difference. Summaries of some recent studies reporting BMD with dual-energy X-ray absorptiometry (DXA) in women with T1DM is shown in table 1.

BONE MINERAL DENSITY STUDIES IN TYPE 2 DIABETES MELLITUS

Several studies have reported higher or similar BMD values women with type 2 diabetes mellitus (T2DM) compared to nondiabetics. Summaries of some studies reporting BMD in diabetic women using DXA is shown in table 2.

Table 1: Bone mineral density in women with type 1 diabetes mellitus with dual-energy X-ray absorptiometry					
Author(s); year	**Country**	**Study population**	**Bone mineral density at different sites in women with or without T1DM**		
			Hip	**Spine**	**Others**
Hadjidakis et al.; 2006	Greece	30 pre-menopausal female patients with T1DM (mean age 32.1 ± 14.8 years) with 30 matched control	Significantly lower in women with T1DM	Similar in both groups	–
Strotmeyer et al.; 2006	United States	67 type 1 diabetic premenopausal women aged 35–55 years and 237 women without diabetes	Lower in women with T1DM	No difference	Lower whole body BMD
Masse et al.; 2016	Canada	27 well-controlled T1DM, and 32 well-matched healthy controls, aged 30–40 years	Significantly decreased in women with T1DM at femur Ward's triangle	Significantly decreased in diabetics	–

T1DM, type 1 diabetes mellitus.

FRACTURE STUDIES

In a population-based study which included 97,090 elderly (> 65 years) women with diabetes and 198,525 women without the disease as control, diabetes increased the risk of fracture: [hazard ratio (HR), 1.11 (1.08–1.15), p <0.0001]. In a meta-analysis of 21 studies involving 82,293 hip fracture events among 6,995,272 participants, diabetes mellitus was associated with an increased risk of hip fractures [relative risk (RR) 2.07; 95% confidence interval (CI) 1.83–2.33]. Excess risk of hip fracture was more pronounced in T1DM (RR 5.76; 95% CI 3.66–9.07) than that in T2DM (RR 1.34; 95% CI 1.19–1.51). Among women with T2DM the excess relative risk of hip fracture was 1.54 (95% CI 1.19–1.99) whereas it was 6.93 (95% CI 4.07–11.78) among women having T1DM.

Women with Type 1 Diabetes Mellitus and Bone Fracture

Women with T1DM were more likely to report a fracture after 20 years of age compared with women without the disease. The Health Improvement Network (THIN) population-based Cohort study from United Kingdom reported that T1DM was associated with increased risk of incident fracture that began in childhood and extended across the lifespan (Table 3). They sustained a disproportionately greater number of lower extremity fractures.

Table 2: Bone mineral density in women with type 2 diabetes mellitus with dual-energy X-ray absorptiometry

Author(s)/year	Country	Study population	Bone mineral density at different sites in women with or without type 2 diabetes mellitus		
			Hip	Spine	Others
Oz et al.; 2006	–	37 females (mean age 54 years) and 34 controls	Significantly higher in cases	No difference	No difference at radius
Yamamoto et al.; 2009	Japan	137 cases (mean age 68 years) and 622 controls	Significantly higher in cases	Significantly higher in cases	Significantly higher at radius in cases
Schwartz et al.; 2013	United States	409 cases (mean age 71 years) and 6,458 control (Study of Osteoporotic Fractures)	Significantly higher in cases but they lost bone more rapidly in controls	Significantly higher in cases but they lost bone more rapidly in controls	–
Leidig-Bruckner et al.; 2014	Germany	128 cases (mean age 63 years) and 249 controls	Significantly higher in cases	Significantly higher in cases	–
Kamalanathan et al.; 2014	India	97 cases and 309 controls	Significantly higher in cases. Not different from BMI-matched control	Significantly higher in cases. Not different from BMI-matched control	–
Mathen et al.; 2015	India	83 cases (mean age 51 years) 87 controls	Significantly lower in cases	Significantly lower in cases	–
Siddapur et al.; 2015	India	30 cases and 30 age-matched (aged 45–75 years)	–	Significantly higher in cases	–
Zhukouskaya et al.; 2015	Italy	99 postmenopausal in good glycemic controls and 107 controls	Significantly higher in cases	Significantly higher in cases	–

Table 3: Studies reporting fracture amongst women with type 1 diabetes mellitus					
Author(s); year	Country	Study population	Fracture rate amongst women with T1DM		Comment
			Hip	Spine	
Miao et al.; 2005	Sweden	12,054 cases (mean age at enrollment 21 years)	After average 9.9 years of follow-up 51 hip fractures	–	Ophthalmic, nephropathic, neurological, and cardiovascular complications were indicators of particularly high risks
Ahmed et al.; 2006	Norway	29 cases and 14,065 controls in Tromsø study	Significantly increased hip fracture risk (RR 8.9, 95% CI 1.2–64.4)	–	–
Janghorbani et al.; 2006	United States	292 cases and 101,343 controls in Nurses' Health study	Age-adjusted RR was 7.1 (95% CI 4.4–11.4)	–	–

T1DM, type 1 diabetes mellitus; RR, relative risk; CI, confidence interval.

Women with Type 2 Diabetes Mellitus and Bone Fracture

The SWAN reported a higher baseline BMD at hip and lumbar spine in diabetics but age-adjusted incident fractures were twofold higher in diabetic women with diabetes compared to those without the disease. Summaries of some studies reporting fracture in T2DM is shown in table 4.

It is notable that DXA which is considered the gold standard for the evaluation of fracture may underestimate the risk. In spite of higher BMD which should indicate increased skeletal strength, women with T2DM are at an increased risk of fracture. The Fracture Risk Assessment Tool (FRAX) score was also another predictor of associated fracture risk. However, for a given T-score and age or FRAX score, participants having diabetes had a higher fracture risk than those without diabetes. The FRAX demonstrated good concordance with observed fractures for general population, but underestimated observed major osteoporotic and hip fracture risk in diabetes. Diabetes confers an increased risk of fracture that is independent of FRAX derived with BMD. This suggested that diabetes might be considered for inclusion in future iterations of FRAX.

QUANTITATIVE COMPUTED TOMOGRAPHY

High-resolution peripheral quantitative computed tomography (HR-pQCT) can characterize microarchitectural and biomechanical abnormalities

Table 4: Studies reporting fracture in type 2 diabetic women

Author(s); year	Country	Study population	Fracture risk amongst women with T2DM		Comment
			Hip	Spine	
Ahmed et al.; 2006	Norway	198 cases and 14,065 controls in Tromsø study	RR 2.0 [95% CI (1.2–3.6)]	–	Increased risk of hip fractures independent of duration of diabetes
Janghorbani et al.; 2006	United States	8,348 cases (mean age 62 years) and 101,343 normal controls in Nurses' Health Study	Age-adjusted RR was 1.7 [95% CI (1.4–2.0)]	–	RRs increased with longer duration of type 2 diabetes [3.1 (2.3–4.0)] for ≥12 years compared with no diabetes and ever use of insulin
Dobnig et al.; 2006	Austria	583 patients with T2DM and 1,081 controls above age 70 years recruited	No significant difference in hip fracture rate of 3.4% among diabetics and 3.1% in controls per 100 patient years	–	–
Bonds et al.; 2006	United States	5,285 cases (mean age 65 years) and 88,120 controls (women without diabetes)	Hip/pelvis/upper leg fracture RR 1.41 (1.17, 1.70)	–	Fracture is occurring despite higher BMD
Yamamoto et al.; 2009	Japan	137 postmenopausal women and 622 controls	–	OR for prevalent vertebral fracture was 1.86 (p = 0.019)	–
Zhukouskaya et al.; 2015	Italy	99 postmenopausal in good glycemic control and 107 controls	–	increased prevalence (34.3%) as compared to controls (18.7%) (p = 0.01)	–

BMD, bone mineral density; RR, relative risk; CI, confidence interval; OR, odds ratio.

using noninvasive, high-resolution three-dimensional imaging. Cortical porosity is significantly higher in subjects with diabetes experiencing fragility fractures when compared with diabetes without fracture. Since DXA is unable to detect these cortical deficits, HR-pQCT could contribute to future fracture risk refinement in subjects with diabetes as well as targeting potential anti-fracture treatments for this population.

DIABETES MEDICATIONS AND BONE HEALTH

Thiazolidinediones (TZDs), therapy results in unbalanced bone remodeling with high bone resorption and low bone formation and consequent bone loss. Health, Aging, and Body Composition observational study demonstrated that each year of TZD use was associated with greater bone loss at the whole body, lumbar spine and trochanter in diabetic women. The Analysis from A Diabetes Outcome Progression Trial (ADOPT) study revealed a twofold increased incidence of bone fracture in women with T2DM treated with rosiglitazone in comparison with other treatment group. Meta-analysis of 10 randomized clinical trials demonstrated increased bone loss at the lumbar spine, total hip, and femoral neck in women on TZD, therapy.

Canagliflozin Cardiovascular Assessment Study (CANVAS) showed significant increase in fractures and was seen with canagliflozin (4.0%) versus placebo (2.6%). Patients in the pooled non-CANVAS studies did not have an increase in fractures with canagliflozin treatment. However, Empagliflozin, Cardiovascular Outcomes, and Mortality in Type 2 Diabetes trial (EMPA-REG OUTCOME) study demonstrated no difference in fracture rates for empagliflozin. There is no evidence for negative effects on bone of other antidiabetes therapies, including biguanides, glucagon-like peptide-1 analogs, and dipeptidyl peptidase-4 inhibitors. Insulin therapy was associated with an increased fracture risk whereas metformin decreased the risk.

MANAGEMENT OF BONE ABNORMALITY IN DIABETES

Glycemic Control and Risk of Fracture

Microvascular complications of diabetes, such as neuropathy, nephropathy, and retinopathy, have been associated with an increased risk of falls and fractures. Additionally, poor glycemic control has been shown to increase fracture risk; however, the fracture benefits of reducing glycosylated hemoglobin (HbA1c) have not been established. In the Action to Control Cardiovascular Risk in Diabetes (ACCORD) randomized trial among individuals with T2DM, neither intensive glycemic control (median HbA1c 6.4% in the intensive group vs. 7.5% in the standard glycemic control group) nor intensive blood pressure control affected the risk of falls or fractures, either positively or negatively.

In T1DM, with intensive insulin therapy weight and BMI increase significantly and correlated with the BMD in the lumbar spine. But patients with diabetic retinopathy continue to lose bone. However, significant hypoglycemia has been associated with increased risk of fall and fracture risk in T2DM.

Lifestyle Interventions

Like in subjects without diabetes, age-appropriate intake of calcium and vitamin D should be ensured in all individuals with diabetes. Weight-bearing physical activity increases bone density in children with T1DM to a degree similar to that in normoglycemic children. Assessment of fall risk and appropriate fall prevention measures should be undertaken in older patients with diabetes.

TREATMENT OF OSTEOPOROSIS IN DIABETES

In women with diabetes, 3 years of alendronate treatment was associated with increased BMD at all sites studied, including 6.6% at the lumbar spine and 2.4% at the hip in the Fracture Intervention Trial (FIT). These changes were similar to normoglycemic individuals. Examination of osteoporosis medication use and fractures in the Danish Registry demonstrated no difference in antifracture efficacy between patients with diabetes and nondiabetic controls or between patients with T1DM and T2DM. Data for strontium usage was limited. In the Raloxifene Use for The Heart (RUTH) trial raloxifene reduced the risk of vertebral fracture risk by 35%, with consistent effects among subgroups including the approximately 4,500 women with diabetes. No definitive data are available for strontium or teriparatide, for which only case reports exist.

CONCLUSION

Fracture risk is increased in individuals with T1DM or T2DM. In T1DM, reduced bone density contributes to fracture risk. In T2DM, BMD is increased in spite of which fracture risk is increased. This indicates that DXA may not be sufficient to assess risk in them. Abnormalities of microarchitectural and biomechanical abnormalities may all contribute, but the precise mechanisms leading to such abnormalities remain unclear. Increased falls due to neuropathy, retinopathy and hypoglycemia also contribute to the higher fracture risk. Improved glycemic control may reduce fracture risk but must be balanced against negative effects of hypoglycemia. Nutrition and lifestyle measures to improve bone health are appropriate for individuals with diabetes, and osteoporosis medications have generally proven to be equally effective in patients with diabetes compared with people without diabetes. Initiation of osteoporosis medications along with adequate calcium and vitamin D supplementation in patients with diabetes with low bone density or low trauma fracture is an appropriate preventive step to maintain bone mineral health.

SUGGESTED READINGS

1. Ahmed LA, Joakimsen RM, Berntsen GK, et al. Diabetes mellitus and the risk of non-vertebral fractures: the Tromsø study. Osteoporos Int. 2006;17:495-500.
2. Bonds DE, Larson JC, Schwartz AV, et al. Risk of fracture in women with type 2 diabetes: the Women's Health Initiative Observational Study. J Clin Endocrinol Metab. 2006;91:3404-10.
3. Dobnig H, Piswanger-Solkner JC, Roth M, et al. Type 2 diabetes mellitus in nursing home patients: effects on bone turnover, bone mass, and fracture risk. J Clin Endocrinol Metab. 2006;91:3355-63.
4. Hadjidakis DJ, Raptis AE, Sfakianakis M, et al. Bone mineral density of both genders in type 1 diabetes according to bone composition. J Diabetes Complications. 2006;20:302-7.
5. Janghorbani M, Feskanich D, Willet WC, et al. Prospective study of diabetes and risk of hip fracture: the Nurses' Health Study. Diabetes Care. 2006;29:1573-8.
6. Kamalanathan S, Nambiar V, Shivane V, et al. Bone mineral density and factors influencing it in Asian Indian population with type 2 diabetes mellitus. Indian J Endocrinol Metab. 2014;18:831-7.
7. Leidig-Bruckner G, Grobholz S, Bruckner T, et al. Prevalence and determinants of osteoporosis in patients with type 1 and type 2 diabetes mellitus. BMC Endocr Disord. 2014;14:33.
8. Masse PG, Pacifique MB, Tranchant CC, et al. Bone metabolic abnormalities associated with well-controlled Type 1 diabetes (IDDM) in young adult women: A disease complication often ignored or neglected. J Am Coll Nutr. 2010;29:419-29.
9. Mathen PG, Thabah MM, Zachariah B, et al. Decreased bone mineral density at the femoral neck and lumbar spine in South Indian patients with type 2 diabetes. J Clin Diagn Res. 2015;9:OC08-12.
10. Miao J, Brismar K, Nyrén O, et al. Elevated hip fracture risk in type 1 diabetic patients: a population-based cohort study in Sweden. Diabetes Care. 2005:28:2850-5.
11. Oz SG, Guven GS, Kilicarslan A, et al. Evaluation of bone metabolism and bone mass in patients with type-2 diabetes mellitus. J Natl Med Assoc. 2006;98:1598-604.
12. Schwartz AV, Ewing SK, Porzig AM, et al. Diabetes and change in bone mineral density at the hip, calcaneus, spine, and radius in older women. Front Endocrinol (Lausanne). 2013;4:62.
13. Siddapur PR, Patil AB, Borde VS. Comparison of Bone Mineral Density, T-Scores and Serum Zinc between Diabetic and non diabetic Postmenopausal Women with Osteoporosis. J Lab Physicians. 2015;7:43-8.
14. Strotmeyer ES, Cauley JA, Orchard TJ, et al. Middle-aged premenopausal women with Type 1 diabetes have lower bone mineral density and calcaneal Quantitative Ultrasound than nondiabetic women. Diabetes Care. 2006;29:306-11.
15. Yamamoto M, Yamaguchi T, Yamauchi M, et al. Diabetic patients have an increased risk of vertebral fractures independent of BMD or diabetic complications. J Bone Miner Res. 2009;24:702-9.
16. Zhukouskaya VV, Eller-Vainicher C, Gaudio A, et al. The utility of lumbar spine trabecular bone score and femoral neck bone mineral density for identifying asymptomatic vertebral fractures in well-compensated type 2 diabetic patients. Osteoporos Int. 2016;27(1):421.

17 CHAPTER

Thyroid Health

KVS Hari Kumar

INTRODUCTION

Thyroid hormones play an essential role in the cellular metabolism and homeostatic functions of the body. The thyroid gland is located in the anterior portion of the neck and secretes thyoxine (T4) and triiodothyronine (T3). Triiodothyronine is the active hormone in the target tissues and is derived mostly from the T4 locally. Thyroid disorders are the second most common endocrine disorders, and are seen in about 5–8% of the population. Diabetes mellitus is a metabolic disorder characterized by the absolute (type 1) or relative (type 2) insulin deficiency and hyperglycemia. Type 2 diabetes mellitus (T2DM) is growing in pandemic proportions and affects about 8–10% of the Indian population. Insulin and thyroid hormones have significant actions in the cellular metabolism and affects the functioning of each other system.

Thyroid disorders have shown to be of increased frequency in the patients with diabetes when compared with the general population. This increased prevalence is due to the advanced age and autoimmunity. About 10% of patients with diabetes have thyroid disorders and the highest prevalence (30%) is seen in females with type 1 diabetes mellitus (T1DM), presumably due to the autoimmune etiology. Autoimmune thyroid disorders (AITD) have been reported more common in females as the sex hormones (estradiol and progesterone) predispose them to autoimmunity. In this chapter, the author has described the etiopathogenic, diagnostic, and therapeutic implications pertaining to the thyroid disorders in women with diabetes. The gender specific issues like gestational diabetes mellitus (GDM) and polycystic ovary syndrome (PCOS) have been described in details with relevant practical points.

THYROID AND DIABETES: BIDIRECTIONAL PATHOPHYSIOLOGICAL LINKS

The Whickham survey published about 4 decades back was the first study that described the link between thyroid dysfunction and diabetes. The bidirectional links between these two endocrinopathies are mediated by the autoimmunity and insulin resistance. Patients with one organ specific autoimmune disease are at risk of developing other autoimmune disorders. Patients with T1DM have higher prevalence of thyroid autoimmunity, thyroid volume, and thyroid dysfunction. Type 1 diabetes mellitus and AITD are common in families and are both mediated by the organ specific T-cell mediated autoimmune attack. The occurrence of T1DM and AITD is known as a polyglandular autoimmune syndrome (PGA) type IIIA. The genetic loci common to both T1DM and AITD include major histocompatibility complex (MHC) locus, *CTLA4, PTPN22, CD25,* etc. The presence of any of these genetic loci doubles the risk of developing either of the disease. The genes involved in linking T2DM with thyroid disorders include *protein kinase B, PEPCK, GLUT-2, and inhibitory G protein.*

Insulin resistance plays a key role in linking the thyroid and diabetes. Thyroid hormones also control the insulin release from the β-cells. Thyroid hormones upregulate the gluconeogenesis and glycogenolysis. Subclinical hypothyroidism has shown to be increasing the risk of insulin resistance through multiple actions on the intracellular actions of the insulin. Insulin resistance is described in both thyroid deficiency and excess states. Thyroid excess results in hepatic insulin resistance whereas the deficiency results in peripheral insulin resistance predominantly. Thyroid hormones promote gluconeogenesis by multiple actions as shown in box 1. Insulin resistance is a common accompaniment of T2DM and diabetes affects the thyroid physiology at multiple levels as shown in box 2.

BOX 1 Effects of thyroid hormones on glucose metabolism

- Promotes gluconeogenesis
- Increases hepatocyte concentration of glucose-6-phosphate
- Increases glucose transporter-2 activity in hepatocytes
- Overproduction of lactate, which is a substrate for gluconeogenesis
- Increased gut glucose absorption
- Increased lipolysis

BOX 2 Effects of diabetes on thyroid physiology

- Central actions
  - Reduced synthesis of TRH
  - Reduced release of TSH
  - Loss of nocturnal peaking effect of TSH
- Peripheral actions
  - Low T3 due to reduced conversion of T4
  - Sick-euthyroid syndrome in marked hyperglycemia
  - Elevated reverse T3
  - Elevated IGF-1 leading to goiter and thyroid nodule development

TRH, thyrotropin releasing hormone; TSH, thyroid stimulating hormone; IGF, insulin-like growth factor; T3, triiodothyronine; T4, thyroxine.

THYROID DYSFUNCTION WITH DIABETES

The spectrum of thyroid disorders in patients with diabetes and their relative frequencies is shown in figure 1. Hypothyroidism and diabetes result in dyslipidemia and have similar risk on the progression of atherosclerotic cardiovascular disease. Subclinical hyperthyroidism may exacerbate the angina and increase the risk for cardiac arrhythmias. Hence, it is essential to screen for the subclinical thyroid dysfunction in patients with diabetes. The complications of diabetes and thyroid disorders exacerbate during their coexistence putting a double trouble for the affected patients. Dysthyroid optic neuropathy is common in diabetics and the microangiopathies of diabetes are common with thyroid dysfunction. Severe diabetic nephropathy mimics hypothyroidism with similar features like edema, pallor, easy fatigability, and weight gain. Sweating, palpitations, and tremulousness are common to both hypoglycemia and hyperthyroidism.

Hypothyroidism results in reduced absorption of the nutrients and often presents with decreasing insulin requirement or with recurrent hypoglycemia. In hypothyroidism, there is reduced insulin secretion

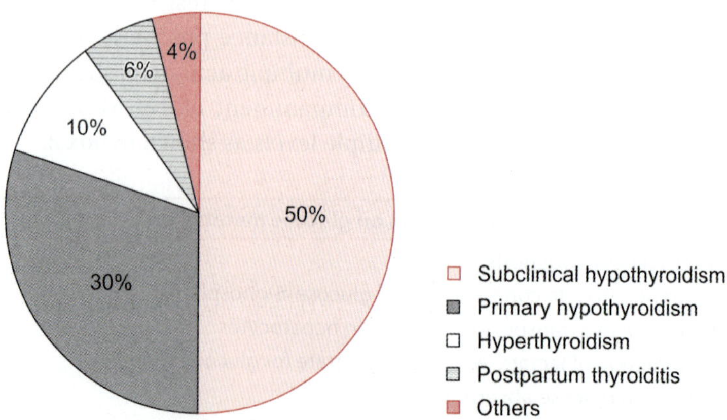

FIG. 1: Prevalence of thyroid disorders in diabetes

and in hyperthyroidism, the β-cell response to glucose is increased. Hyperthyroidism is associated with an increase in the insulin requirement and worsening glycemic control. There is increased hepatic gluconeogenesis, rapid gastrointestinal glucose absorption, and increase in the insulin resistance. It may unmask the latent diabetes in individuals. Insulin clearance is increased in thyrotoxicosis leading to reduced action. "Thyroid diabetes" denotes the diabetes resulting from thyroid hormone excess leading to an increase in the insulin requirement. The summary of the clinical, diagnostic, and therapeutic aspects of thyroid dysfunction in diabetes is given in table 1.

Table 1: Salient features of thyroid dysfunction in diabetes

Feature	Hypothyroidism	Hyperthyroidism
Patho-physiology	• Reduced nutrient absorption • Reduced insulin secretion • Prolonged insulin half-life • Reduced peripheral utilization of glucose • Reduced hepatic glucose output • Impaired muscle glycogenolysis	• Increased gluconeogenesis and glycogenolysis • Rapid gastrointestinal absorption • Reduced insulin half-life • Increased insulin clearance
Net effect	• Hypoglycemia	• Hyperglycemia
Clinical features	• Edema, pallor, and easy fatigability • Mimics diabetic nephropathy	• Weight loss, catabolic state may mimic diabetic ketoacidosis • Tachycardia, sweating, and tremors are common symptoms of hypoglycemia and hyperthyroidism
Investi-gations	• Low T3 and T4 due to protein loss in diabetic nephropathy • Spurious elevation of HbA1c due to low red blood cells turnover	• Low T3 and T4 may be pseudonormal in severe hyperglycemia and may delay the diagnosis of hyperthyroidism • Abnormal response to glucose tolerance test due to faster absorption of glucose • Hyperthyroidism may unmask the latent diabetes
Manage-ment	• Reduced requirements of oral hypoglycemic agents/ insulin • Metformin reduces thyroid stimulating hormone level	• Increased requirement of oral hypoglycemic agents or insulin

T3, triiodothyronine; T4, thyoxine; HbA1c, glycated hemoglobin.

THYROID DISORDERS WITH GESTATIONAL DIABETES MELLITUS AND POLYCYSTIC OVARY SYNDROME

The risk of GDM and postpartum thyroiditis is more in patients with AITD. The prevalence of thyroid autoantibodies is seen about 10–20% of pregnant women with GDM. Gestational diabetes mellitus has been shown to affect the expression of the thyroid hormone transporters like monocarboxylate transporter 8 and monocarboxylate transporter 10 in the placenta. The presence of thyroid autoantibodies induces the release of proinflammatory cytokines, which augment the insulin resistance. Inflammatory mediators, including C-reactive protein are the main links between the AITD and the insulin resistance. Patients with PCOS have also been reported to have a higher prevalence of thyroid disorders, including subclinical hypothyroidism and AITD. Estrogen is a potent immune enhancer and the women with PCOS have a characteristically high estrogen to progesterone ratio. Progesterone usually counteracts the immune enhancing effect of the estrogen. However, in patients with PCOS, the relatively low concentration of progesterone is unable to reduce this immunogenicity. The high levels of luteinizing hormone in PCOS stimulate the estrogen, which stimulates the thyroid gland through thyroid stimulating hormone (TSH).

THYROID CANCER AND DIABETES

Obesity and diabetes have been shown to be associated with increased risk of differentiated thyroid cancer (DTC). Insulin directly contributes to the growth of thyroid cancer cells by stimulating the insulin like growth factor-1 (IGF-1) receptor. The IGF-1 receptor activates the mitogen-activated protein kinase and phosphoinositide 3-kinase pathways which regulate the gene expression, differentiation, and mitosis. Patients with diabetes have increased visceral fat, where the aromatase enzyme converts testosterone to estradiol. The relative excess of estradiol promotes the malignant transformation of the thyroid follicular cells. The high prevalence of DTC is also mediated by the leptin in obese people. Leptin promotes cell proliferation, inhibits apoptosis, promotes angiogenesis, tumor invasion, and also promotes the pituitary production of the TSH. Thyroid stimulating hormone stimulates the adenylate cyclase, cyclic adenosine monophosphate (AMP) protein kinase A system that regulates the differentiation and proliferation of the thyroid gland. The protein kinase C system led to activation of the certain oncogenes, thereby, promoting the cancer progression. The oxidative stress is a proinflammatory condition leading to the release of free radicals, tumor necrosis factor-α, and reactive oxygen species and malignant transformation of the thyroid follicular

BOX 3	Mechanisms of increased thyroid cancer in diabetes

- High insulin which is a growth factor for follicular epithelium
- Increased insulin-like growth factor-1
- Mild elevated thyroid stimulating hormone levels
- Increased leptin
- Oxidative stress
- Proinflammatory cytokine release
- Vitamin D deficiency
- Reduced expression of the type 2 iodothyronine deiodinase enzyme

cells. The type 2 iodothyronine deiodinase enzyme (DIO2) regulates the intracellular thyroid hormone levels and also the expression of the *GLUT-4*. Deficiency of this leads to insulin resistance and increased risk of thyroid malignancy. The various mechanisms involved in increased risk of thyroid cancer in diabetes are summarized in box 3.

MANAGEMENT OF THYROID DISORDERS IN DIABETES

The coexistence of the thyroid disorders would increase the healthcare burden in patients with diabetes. The delay in identification of the underlying thyroid disorders often leads to poor management of the diabetes. Hence, the treating physicians have to be aware about the need to screen for thyroid disorders as shown in box 4. The management of thyroid disorders remains the same in patients with or without diabetes. However, certain peculiarities exist in patients with diabetes. The management of the thyroid condition always leads to the change in the glycemic control and the practitioners have to be more dynamic in anticipating the change and take the necessary remedial steps in reducing the morbidity. Levothyroxine replacement therapy may exacerbate the myocardial ischemia in patients with diabetes and hypothyroidism. Hence, a gradual replacement is necessary with an increment of 25 µg every month or alternate months. Thyroxine replacement therapy should be offered to diabetes patients with subclinical hypothyroidism, if they have dyslipidemia, goiter, and positive thyroid antibodies.

BOX 4	When to screen for thyroid disorders?

- Recurrent hypoglycemia
- Unexplained hypoglycemia
- Reducing requirement of insulin/oral hypoglycemic agents
- Unexplained weight change
- Persisting dyslipidemia
- Unexplained changes in glycemic control

BOX 5	Mechanisms of metformin-induced thyroid dysfunction

- Reduction in the thyroid stimulating hormone levels
- Change in the number and affinity of the thyroid receptors
- Increased gastrointestinal absorption of the L-thyroxine
- Change in the thyroid hormone protein binding
- Altered thyroid hormone metabolism
- Interference in the thyrotropin assay
- Antimitogenic activity and reduces thyroid cancer
- Reduced goiter and thyroid nodule size

Hyperthyroidism worsens the underlying diabetic state and early definitive therapy using the radioiodine or surgery may be considered instead of prolonged use of antithyroid drugs (ATDs). The remission rate with the use of ATDs is even less in diabetes, when compared with nondiabetic patients. Patients with toxic multinodular goiter and solitary toxic nodule should be offered early surgery as the untreated thyrotoxicosis also exacerbates the cardiac ischemia in patients with diabetes. The thyroid suppressive therapy in patients with DTC may worsen the preexisting diabetes. However, it is recommended to uptitrate the antidiabetic medications and not under replace the thyroxine to prevent the recurrence of the malignancy. In patients with PGA, the use of multiple medications like thyroxine, glucocorticoids, estrogen, and progesterone may affect the glycemic control.

Metformin is a commonly used oral antidiabetic drug and has multiple effects on the thyroid. The use of metformin results in reduction of the TSH levels without any significant changes in the thyroid hormones. The observed changes are mediated by the altered dopaminergic regulation of thyrotropin secretion and are reduced with the use of bromocriptine. The mechanisms of metformin-induced thyroid dysfunction have been summarized in box 5. Metformin activates the peripheral AMP-activated protein kinase (AMPK) pathway, but inhibits the hypothalamic AMPK pathway. Metformin has been recommended in patients with amiodarone-induced hypothyroidism who are intolerant to the T4 replacement.

GUIDELINES AND PRACTICE POINTS

There are no formal guidelines from the endocrine or thyroid societies about the management of thyroid disorders in women with diabetes. They have published a consensus statement in 2005 regarding the screening for thyroid dysfunction in patients with diabetes as shown in flowchart 1. Few studies have shown a significant yield with routine screening, whereas, few population studies have shown that the prevalence is not high that warrant a routine screening. A high index of clinical suspicion is required in difficult to treat diabetes cases to identify the thyroid abnormality as shown in box 6.

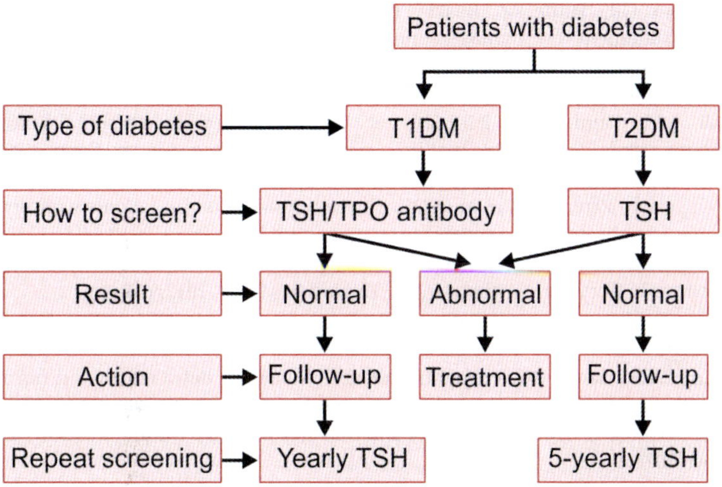

T1DM, type 1 diabetes mellitus; T2DM, type 2 diabetes mellitus; TSH, thyroid stimulating hormone; TPO, thyroid peroxidase.

FLOWCHART 1: Screening for thyroid disorders in diabetes

BOX 6 Clinical pearls in thyroid with diabetes

- Be cautious in diagnosing diabetes during hyperthyroidism
- Look for hyperthyroidism in diabetes patients with unexplained hyperglycemia
- Be dynamic in adjusting the antidiabetic drugs during thyroid dysfunction
- Look for hypothyroidism in patients with reducing antidiabetic drug requirement
- Look for hypopituitarism in hypothyroidism patients with reducing insulin requirement

CONCLUSION

To conclude, the thyroid disorders are common in patients with diabetes with profound implications on the glycemic and metabolic control. Regular screening is indicated for early detection and definitive management of subclinical thyroid dysfunction. Management of thyroid disorders is similar to nondiabetic patients with certain peculiarities.

CONFLICT OF INTEREST

The author declares that he has no conflict of interest.

SUGGESTED READINGS

1. Demitrost L, Ranabir S. Thyroid dysfunction in type 2 diabetes mellitus: A retrospective study. Indian J Endocrinol Metab. 2012;16:S334-5.
2. Duntas LH, Orgiazzi J, Brabant G. The interface between thyroid and diabetes mellitus. Clin Endocrinol (Oxf). 2011;75(1):1-9.

3. Hossein GR, Tuttle M, Baskin HJ, et al. Subclinical thyroid dysfunction: a joint statement on management from the American Association of Clinical Endocrinologists, the American Thyroid Association, and the Endocrine Society. J Clin Endocrinol Metab. 2005;90:581-5.
4. Jali MV, Kambar S, Jali SM, et al. Prevalence of thyroid dysfunction among type 2 diabetes mellitus patients. Diabetes Metab Syndr. 2016;pii: S1871-4021(16)30260-0.
5. Kadiyala R, Peter R, Okosieme OE. Thyroid dysfunction in patients with diabetes: clinical implications and screening strategies. Int J Clin Pract. 2010;64(8):1130-9.
6. Kalra S, Kalra B, Chatley G. Prevalence of hypothyroidism in pediatric type 1 diabetes mellitus in Haryana, Northern India. Thyroid Res Pract. 2012;9:12-4.
7. Kalra S, Unnikrishnan AG, Sahay R. The hypoglycemic side of hypothyroidism. Indian J Endocrinol Metab. 2014;18(1):1-3.
8. Kumar HK, Yadav RK, Prajapati J, et al. Association between thyroid hormones, insulin resistance, and metabolic syndrome. Saudi Med J. 2009;30(7):907-11.
9. Ray S, Ghosh S. Thyroid disorders and diabetes mellitus: Double trouble. J Dia Res Ther. 2016;2(1).
10. Wu P. Thyroid disease and diabetes. Clinical Diabetes. 2000;18:38-9

18

CHAPTER

Eating Disorders

Mudita Dhingra, Bharti Kalra

INTRODUCTION

Diabetes is associated with increased risk of a number of eating disorders. Some of these are more frequently associated with a particular type of diabetes than others. Binge eating disorder, for instance, is more common in patients with type 2 diabetes mellitus (T2DM).

Type 1 diabetes mellitus (T1DM) is a chronic condition characterized by absolute insulin deficiency whereas T2DM is a metabolic disease, primarily characterized by insulin resistance.

The aim of diabetes treatment is to normalize blood glucose level with the help of diet, moderate exercise, and medications in form of insulin or oral antidiabetics and insulin and supply of cells. Eating disorders are disorders of eating behaviors, associated thoughts, attitudes, and emotions, and their resulting psychological impairment. Anorexia nervosa and bulimia nervosa are the major eating disorders that are included in Diagnostic and Statistical Manual of Mental Disorders, 4th edition. Anorexia nervosa is further classified into binge eating/purging type and restricting type. Bulimia nervosa is also divided into purging and nonpurging type. In addition to the above classification, International Classification of Diseases, 10th revision, also includes atypical anorexia nervosa, atypical bulimia nervosa, vomiting associated with other psychological disturbance, and overeating associated with other psychological disturbances. Another category for patients who do not fit into particular category is eating disorders otherwise not specified (EDNOS). Eating disorders associated with diabetes may include insulin omission/dose reduction, and dietary manipulation. Eating disorders are poorly understood and underdiagnosed aspect of diabetes management. More holistic approach and team effort is needed for appropriate biomedical outcome.

DEFINITION

An eating disorder is a serious mental health issue that involves preoccupation with control over one's body weight, shape, eating, and exercise.

There are four main types of eating disorders:

1 Anorexia nervosa
2 Bulimia nervosa
3 Binge eating disorders
4 Eating disorders not otherwise specified.

Anorexia Nervosa

- Severe restriction of food intake
- Loss of body weight to an unhealthy level
- Secondary amenorrhea/oligomenorrhea
- Losing control of eating.

Bulimia Nervosa

- Repeated episodes of overeating (1–2/week over 3 months)—large amount of food consumed in short time
- Persistent preoccupation with eating and craving for food
- Attempts to compensate for weight gain one or more of the following method: Self-induced vomiting, self-induced purging, alternating with periods of starvation or use of drugs, e.g., diuretics
- Self-perception of being too fat.

Binge Eating Disorder

- Repeated episodes of binge eating without compensatory behavior
- Eating when not hungry and eating until uncomfortably full
- It is associated with increased psychopathology including depression and personality disorders

Eating Disorders not Otherwise Specified

Eating disorders not fitting into above mentioned categories are discussed in this category.

Young women with diabetes have more than double the risk of developing an eating disorder than women without diabetes. It can affect up to 20% of females with diabetes.

It is also common in young people with diabetes to manipulate insulin dosage in order to manage their body weight. It is defined as diabulimia.

Eating disorders are ego-syntonic in nature, which means the patients view eating disorders as a solution to their problems, and therefore, the diagnosis is delayed. Most of the studies that report prevalence of these disorders are questionnaire based, and therefore, may not represent true occurrence. Disordered eating behavior is often well-hidden; women with diabetes should be encouraged to discuss a range of weight related issues.

Healthcare providers should be vigilant for symptoms of eating disorders and develop validated screening tool which can help in early recognition. If left untreated, this disorder can increase risk of retinopathy threefold and even premature death.

Not only T1DM but also T2DM children are prone to eating disorders, particularly binge eating disorder. Whereas, intentional omission of insulin doses for the purpose of weight loss occurs mainly in patient with T1DM, in patients with T2DM, omission of oral hypoglycemic drugs can be present.

PATHOPHYSIOLOGY

There are two models proposed for pathophysiology of eating disorders in diabetes mellitus:

1. Daneman et al. developed a model to describe hypotheses for the link between T1DM and abnormal eating or weight-related behaviors. According to this model, insulin therapy may trigger eating disorders, as it causes an increase in weight. This increase in weight can cause body dissatisfaction and a drive for thinness, which can lead to so-called "restrained eating behavior" (dieting), interrupted by recurring attacks of eating (Fig. 1)
2. Three level model to describe the development of disturbed eating in adolescent with T1DM.

First circle: Premorbid status, increased body weight, and tendency to gain weight.

Asking simple questions to an adolescent girl like "Have you ever been overweight?" may be helpful in screening patients who are at high risk of eating disorders. Family characteristics and dynamics are also associated with higher prevalence of eating disorders. Families where parents tend to

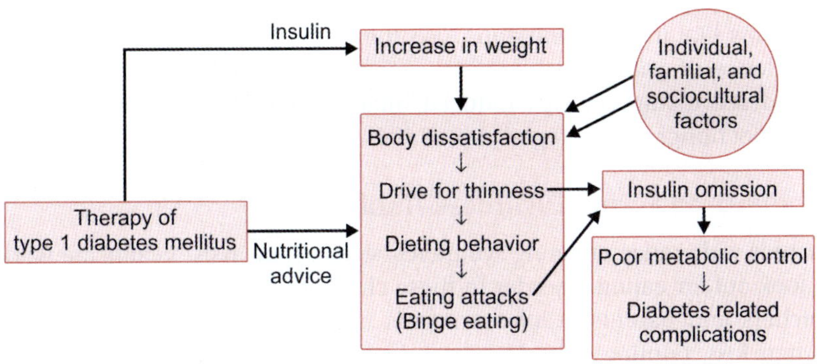

FIG 1: Model for the connections between type 1 diabetes mellitus and eating disorders

make negative comments about weight/eating and mothers who themselves indulge in binge eating and dieting are more likely to have daughters with eating disorders. Personality characteristics also contribute to occurrence of eating disorders. Adolescent girls with T1DM and eating disorders show deficit in self-regulation and narcissistic gain. Similarly, borderline personality characteristics were associated with insulin omission.

Second circle: It includes factors associated with disease onset. Age at diagnosis of diabetes mellitus plays a crucial role in occurrence of eating disorder (higher prevalence in 7–18 years age group). Thus, the development of T1DM in preadolescent and adolescent age places these girls at increased risk of anorexia nervosa and bulimia nervosa. Frequent omission/reduction of dosage of insulin was reported in these age groups as these children often do not like their parents to involve in day-to-day management.

Third circle: It includes factors associated with chronic management of diabetes like intensive insulin regimen, dietary restraints (results in craving and binge eating of "forbidden foods"), frequency of hypoglycemic episodes (accompanied by intense hunger, especially for sweet foods), and psychological illness including depression.

Risk Factors

- Female gender
- Large fluctuations in body weight, e.g., reduction in weight at diagnosis of diabetes and increase after starting insulin
- Higher body mass index
- Depressed mood and low self-esteem (particularly in T2DM)
- Disturbed family function.

DIAGNOSIS

Diagnosis of eating disorder in T1DM is challenging as it is often hidden or denied. Standard questionnaires made for diagnosis of eating disorders cannot be applied to children with diabetes as they do not recognize specific problems like insulin omission. Also these questionnaires may inflate the prevalence of eating problems in such children as behaviors which are considered disturbed, e.g., reduced intake of certain food groups, eating when not hungry, are integral part of diabetes care.

Recognizing Eating Disorders (Table 1)

There is wide range of eating symptoms/signs which assist healthcare worker to look out for eating disorder in these children. It can even be reported by teachers and parents. Adolescent girls may complain of symptoms such as hair loss, fainting episodes, or abdominal pain but are unlikely to give information about dieting or omitting insulin.

Table 1: Recognizing eating disorders in diabetes	
Psychosocial influences	• Deterioration in psychological functioning, e.g., relationship with peers • Avoid eating with family and peers
Diabetes management	• Self-critical thoughts • Preoccupation with food or meal planning • Low mood, anxiety, or irritability • Obsessive calorie and carbohydrate counting
Cognitive factors	• Poor attendance at clinic • Increased concern about body shape or weight • Poor metabolic control despite appearance of compliance
Physical factors	• General symptom: Weight gain/weight loss • Dermatological: Thin hair , pale dry skin, puffy face, feeling cold • Metabolic features: Repeated diabetic ketoacidosis, electrolyte abnormality, e.g., hypokalemia, hypoglycemia • Cardiovascular: Hypotension, tachycardia, dizziness, and fainting • Gastrointestinal: Abdominal pain, irritable bowel syndrome, or constipation
Behavioral factors	• Going to bathroom after eating • Avoiding eating with others • Cooking for others but not eating • Reading diet magazines, articles, and watching food related programs

Red Flag Signs

- Changes in eating habits (eating more but still losing weight)
- Unexplained weight loss
- Unexplained high blood sugar
- Low energy levels
- Frequent urination.

TYPE 2 DIABETES MELLITUS AND EATING DISORDERS

The Treatment options for Type 2 Diabetes in Adolescent and Youth (TODAY) trial studied 678 children (64.9% girls) with T2DM (mean age 14.0 years;) proved that youth with clinical (6%) and subclinical (20%) levels of binge eating had significantly higher levels and rates of extreme obesity, global eating disorder, and depressive symptoms with impaired quality of life. The presence of binge eating in youth with T2DM is particularly troubling given the association of binge eating with accelerated weight gain in those who are already overweight.

COMPLICATIONS

Short-term complications:

- Repeated episodes of severe hypoglycemia
- Diabetic ketoacidosis (DKA)
- Prolonged hospital stay.

Long-term complications:

- Hypertension
- Dyslipidemia
- Retinopathy (increase threefold)
- Nephropathy
- Premature death.

Mortality rates per 1,000 person/year:

- About 2.2 in girls with T1DM
- About 7.3 in girls with eating disorder
- About 34.6 in girls with both eating disorder and T1DM.

PREVENTION

Promoting the understanding and awareness among healthcare providers of factors involved in the development of eating disorders in young vulnerable individuals with T1DM may help prevent these disorders. These factors include weight gain with the initiation of insulin treatment, the dietary restraint necessitated by diabetes management, and recurrent hypoglycemic episodes. Therefore, flexible approach in diabetes management should be promoted. Interventions aimed at increasing self-esteem and body acceptance, as well as family-based interventions aimed to improve family management of obesity and diabetes may also help to diminish the risk of developing eating disorders. Brief interactive programs and support group can also help in reducing development of eating disorders in adolescent girls.

MANAGEMENT

It is often complex and difficult to treat the cycle of negative feelings about body shape and image in young women with already coexisting chronic illness.

Goals:

- Attaining and maintaining a normal, healthy, individualized, stable body weight
- Stopping all abnormal eating behaviors, such as food restricting, binge eating, or purging, and associated abnormal behaviors, especially compulsive exercise

- Dismantling the core overvalued beliefs and unhealthy cognitive "schemas" of automatic cognitive distortions, replacing them with healthy, balanced views of self (not primarily dependent on body weight or shape), and the capacity for emotional and behavioral self-regulation
- Treating the comorbid conditions, psychiatric and medical
- Planning for ongoing relapse prevention for approximately 5 years after acute improvement.

Early treatment is important because the longer an eating disorder continues, the harder it is to treat. Treatment includes decreasing dietary restraints, promoting healthy eating, and psychological interventions to address underlying psychopathology. The treatment of choice is family therapy. Minimally this should include a psychologist, a specialist eating disorder dietician, and a psychotherapist. Families and healthcare providers are essential members of the treatment team. Close physical monitoring should be maintained and therapeutic support for changing thoughts and behaviors is encouraged.

CONCLUSION

Eating disorders commonly coexist with diabetes, and if not identified early, they can lead to serious and accelerated complications, particularly retinopathy. Young women with diabetes have more than double the risk of developing an eating disorder than women without diabetes. About one-third of individuals with T1DM intentionally omit insulin. Diagnosis of eating disorders in individuals with T1DM is difficult, since eating disorder behaviors are often well-hidden. Weight loss that is related to deteriorated glycemic control and recurrent DKA should raise suspicion. Early diagnosis is essential, occurrence of eating disorders and diabetes together is associated with increased morbidity and mortality. If eating disorder is suspected, child should be referred to a mental health counselor who is specialized in eating disorders. A strong collaboration between psychologist and diabetes care provider can help avoid secondary physical and psychological diseases. Above all, support from family, uninterrupted communications among family members, mother's positive attitude towards body image represent factors for successful treatment. However, further research is warranted to study this often ignored concurrent problem of eating disorder in young woman with diabetics.

SUGGESTED READINGS

1. Daneman D, Olmsted M, Rydall A, et al. Eating disorders in young women with type 1 diabetes. Prevalence, problems and prevention. Horm Res. 1998;50(Suppl 1):79-86.
2. Daneman D, Rodin G, Jones J. Eating disorders in adolescent girls and young adult women with type 1 diabetes. Diabetes Spectrum. 2002;15:83-105.

3. Diagnostic and statistical manual of mental disorders. 5th edition. Washington DC: American Psychiatric Association; 2013.
4. Philpot U. Eating disorders in young people: development, diagnosis and management. J Diabetes Nurs. 2013;17(6):228-32.
5. Pinhas-Hamiel O, Hamiel U, Levy-Shraga Y, et al. Eating disorders in adolescents with type 1 diabetes: Challenges in diagnosis and treatment. World J Diabetes. 2015 April;6(3):517-26.
6. Racicka E, Brynska A. Eating disorders in children and adolescents with type 1 and type 2 diabetes—prevalence , risk factor®s , warning signs. Psychiatr Pol. 2015;49(5):1017-24.
7. Sharan P, Sundar AS. Eating disorders in women. Indian J Psychiatry. 2015;57:286-95.
8. The ICD-10 Classification of Mental and Behavioral Disorders. Diagnostic Criteria for Research. Geneva: World Health Organization; 1993.

19
CHAPTER

Contraception

Beena Bansal, Parjeet Kaur

INTRODUCTION

A 31-year-old female visited endocrinology outpatient department for management of diabetes. She has been married for last 4 years and gave birth to a baby boy 18 months back. She was diagnosed to have gestational diabetes mellitus during her 24 weeks of period of gestation. Blood glucose normalized after delivery and subsequently she did not check her glucose levels. Two months back she was diagnosed to have type 2 diabetes mellitus (T2DM) and was put on oral antidiabetes drugs. However, her glycemic control was not good. Her main concerns were adverse effects of medications during lactation and pregnancy planning in future. She was already apprehensive about contraception because of cultural taboos and fear of worsening of glycemic control with use of contraceptives. This case highlights the need of educating women with diabetes about significant role of contraception and various contraceptives options available to achieve a good prepregnancy glycemic control. Achieving a good glycemic control prior to conception is a challenge faced by many healthcare professionals, as many women with diabetes do not plan their pregnancy. A United States national survey found that women with diabetes were less likely to be using contraception than women without diabetes. This problem is expected to be even worse in India due to various reasons such as social taboo, lack of understanding of risk of poor glycemic control in pregnancy, lack of knowledge of contraceptive choices, and hesitation in discussing contraception with healthcare providers.

A CRUCIAL ROLE FOR CONTRACEPTION IN DIABETIC WOMEN

Despite the fact that unplanned pregnancies are fraught with maternal and fetal complications, the use of contraception has been reported to be lower in women with diabetes as compared to those without diabetes. This may be related to the fear of cardiovascular complications with the use of hormone-based contraception. However, this risk has to be balanced with the risk of unplanned pregnancies. Unplanned pregnancy can be harmful both to diabetic mother as well as her offspring. Diabetic mother with poor glycemic control is prone to increased risk of hypertension and preeclampsia, as well as the worsening of preexisting degenerative complications such as retinopathy or nephropathy. Fetal complications include increased risk of congenital abnormalities, spontaneous abortion, *in utero* death, fetal overgrowth leading to macrosomia, neonatal hypoglycemia, and hyperbilirubinemia. Hence, it is important to discuss the pros and cons of various contraceptive methods to enable informed choice in these women.

OVERVIEW OF CONTRACEPTIVE CHOICES

Contraceptive choices can be broadly divided into hormonal contraception and nonhormonal contraception (Box 1). Hormonal contraceptive methods are further divided into long-term methods—intrauterine devices (IUDs) and long-acting progestin only contraceptives (POC) methods, and short-term methods—combined oral contraceptives (COCs), nonoral combination hormonal methods which can be administered as a monthly injection, a transdermal patch, or an intravaginal ring, daily progestin oral contraceptive and emergency contraception. Nonhormonal contraceptive methods include male and female condoms, diaphragms, caps, shields, spermicides, withdrawal, fertility awareness, and natural family planning. At the completion of childbearing, elective sterilization may be considered.

BOX 1 Contraception choices for women with diabetes

Hormonal contraceptive methods

- Long-term methods
  - Intrauterine devices
  - Long-acting progestin-only contraceptives methods
- Short-term methods
  - Combined oral contraceptives
  - Nonoral combination hormonal methods
  - Daily progestin oral contraceptive
  - Emergency contraception

Nonhormonal contraceptive methods

- Barrier methods
  - Condoms, diaphragms, cervical caps, and spermicides

INTRAUTERINE DEVICES

Intrauterine devices include copper IUD and levonorgestrel intrauterine system (LNG IUS). Both are effective methods of contraception, with a failure rate of less than 1%. They are safe because no increased risk of pelvic inflammatory diseases have been demonstrated even in diabetic women. The risk of bleeding is low in LNG IUS. The release of hormone from it being quite low, no effect on lipids or glycemia has been shown in women using LNG IUS. A systematic review on the efficacy of the IUD and IUS for women with diabetes mellitus found that copper IUD and LNG IUS were suitable for women with type 1 diabetes mellitus and T2DM.

Long-acting Progestin-only Contraceptive Methods

Intramuscular Implant

Depomedroxyprogesterone acetate (DMPA): This is the most common type of injectable contraceptive. It is given in a dose of 150 mg intramuscularly every 3 months. It is marketed as "Depo-Provera" in India.

Norethindrone enanthate (NET-EN): It is given in a dose of 200 mg intramuscularly every 2 months. Currently, it is not available in India.

The advantages of long-acting POC methods are that they are very effective, long-acting, and reversible. Disadvantages include:

- Changes in menstrual bleeding pattern, like irregular spotting or bleeding, scanty periods are common, rarely heavy bleeding may occur. Amenorrhea, especially after 1st year of use, may be disturbing in some women
- Return of fertility may take up to 9 months after the last injection which is longer than other reversible contraceptive methods
- Greater weight gain
- Unfavorable effects on lipids and glucose due to hypoestrogenic effects. Depomedroxyprogesterone acetate in several studies has shown more adverse effects on lipids and insulin resistance compared with minimal effects of norplant.

Subcutaneous Implant

- Norplant, with six levonorgestrel rods lasting 5 years; neutral on lipids and glucose
- Implanon, with one etonogestrel rod; lasting 3 years.

Progestin-only subcutaneous implants are better suited for women with diabetes compared to intramuscular implants due to constant release of progestogen dose maintaining steady blood lipid ratios.

Combined Oral Contraceptives

Combined oral contraceptives combine ethinylestradiol (EE) in various doses with second generation (levonorgestrel or norgestimate) and third generation (desogestrel and gestodene) progestins.

Ethinylestradiol is added to improve cycle control. The metabolic effects of EE include:

- No effect on glucose levels or insulin sensitivity
- Increase in risk of thrombosis because of its effect on hemostasis
- Increase in triglyceride and high density lipoprotein (HDL) cholesterol level, decrease in low density lipoprotein (LDL) cholesterol
- Increase in blood pressure because of effect on renin-angiotensin system.

Hence, lowest possible dose of EE should be prescribed in women with T2DM.

The metabolic effects of progestins include:

- Decrease in insulin sensitivity
- No effect on clotting
- No effect on blood pressure
- Decrease in triglyceride and HDL cholesterol, increase in LDL cholesterol.

Clinically this translates into:

- Increased risk of myocardial infarction (MI) at least by twofolds. The risk is seen especially with second generation progestins. It is increased if other risk factors for MI are present like hypertension, smoking, family history of cardiac events, and diabetes. Patients with hypertension have 16- to 58-fold increased risk of MI with COC use
- Increased risk of thrombosis with both generations of COCs. Patients with migraine have two- to fourfold increased risk of thrombosis. The risk of thrombosis increases with increasing dose of EE and does not depend on the type of progestin.

Nonoral Combination Hormonal Methods

- Monthly injection
- Transdermal patch
- Vaginal ring.

The risks or benefits of nonoral hormonal methods are less well-studied but appear similar to oral methods.

Barrier Methods

Barrier methods including condoms, diaphragms, spermicides, and cervical caps are safe because they do not have any systemic metabolic effects. They also help in prevention of sexually transmitted diseases. However, the failure rates are unacceptably high at 20%. This has to be addressed by adequate patient and partner counseling in case there are contraindications to other contraceptive methods.

DISCUSSING DIABETES, PREGNANCY, AND BIRTH CONTROL WITH WOMEN

The significance of avoiding unplanned pregnancy should be discussed by doctors and diabetes educators from adolescence onward and should be an integral part of diabetes education. Selection of a contraceptive method must take into account the woman's preferences, her time frame for pregnancy, and contraceptive efficacy, safety, and side effects. Options of various contraceptives should be discussed in detail with woman including risks and benefits of each option. Carefully chosen, safe, and reliable method of contraception for a woman with diabetes is vital, and practitioners should refer to World Health Organization Medical Eligibility Criteria for Contraceptive Use (Table 1).

Table 1: World Health Organization Medical Eligibility Criteria for Contraceptive use

Condition	CHC	POP	DMPA/ NET-EN	IMP	Cu IUD	IUS
History of gestational diabetes	1	1	1	1	1	1
Type 2 diabetes mellitus	2	2	2	2	1	2
Type 1 diabetes mellitus	2	2	2	2	1	2
Neuropathy/nephropathy/retinopathy	3/4	2	3	2	1	2
Other vascular disease or diabetes >20 years duration	3/4	2	3	2	1	2

WHO Medical Eligibility Criteria for Contraceptive Use (2015)

1 = No restriction for the use of this method.

2 = Advantages of using the method generally outweigh the theoretical or proven risks.

3 = Theoretical or proven risks usually outweigh the advantages of using the method.

4 = Unacceptable health risk.

CHC, combined hormonal contraception; Cu IUD, copper intrauterine device; DMPA/NET-EN, depot medroxyprogesterone acetate/norethisterone enanthate; IMP, implants; POP, progestogen-only pill; IUS, intrauterine system.

Source: WHO. WHO Medical Eligibility Criteria for Contraceptive Use; Geneva: 2015. [online] Available from: http://www.who.int/reproductivehealth/publications/family_planning/mec-wheel-5th/en/ (10). (Accessed April, 2017).

CONCLUSION

In females with T2DM, IUDs are effective and safe to use in all females. Both copper IUD and LNG IUS are safe, while risk of bleeding is lower with LNG IUS. Combined oral contraceptives can be given in females with T2DM, but should be avoided in those more than 40 years of age, hypertensive, having family history of cardiac events, migraine, or history of smoking. Third generation COCs should be preferred because the risk of MI and thrombosis being low with them. Nonoral hormonal contraception and POPs have similar side effect profile as oral COCs, and can be used when compliance is an issue. At the completion of childbearing, elective sterilization may be considered.

SUGGESTED READINGS

1. Crook D, Godsland I. Safety evaluation of modern oral contraceptives. Effects on lipoprotein and carbohydrate metabolism. Contraception. 1998;57:189-201.
2. Goldstuck ND, Steyn PS. The intrauterine device in women with diabetes mellitus type I and II: a systematic review. ISRN Obstet Gynecol. 2013;2013:81406.
3. Kahn HS, Curtis KM, Marchbanks PA. Effects of injectable or implantable progestin-only contraceptives on insulinglucose metabolism and diabetes risk. Diabetes Care. 2003;26:216-25.
4. Kim C, Siscovick DS, Sidney S, et al. Oral contraceptive use and association with glucose, insulin, and diabetes in young adult women: the CARDIA Study. Coronary Artery Risk Development in Young Adults. Diabetes Care. 2002;25:1027-32.
5. Lopez LM, Grimes DA, Schulz KF. Steroidal contraceptives: effect on carbohydrate metabolism in women without diabetes mellitus. Cochrane Database Syst Rev. 2007:CD006133.
6. O'Brien SH, Koch T, Vesely SK, et al. Hormonal Contraception and Risk of Thromboembolism in Women With Diabetes. Diabetes Care. 2017;40(2):233-8.
7. Pregnancy outcomes in the Diabetes Control and Complications Trial. American Journal of Obstetrics and Gynecology. 1996;174:1343-53.
8. Vahratian A, Barber JS, Lawrence JM, et al. Family-planning practices among women with diabetes and overweight and obese women in the 2002 National Survey for Family Growth. Diabetes Care. 2009;32:1026-31.
9. World Health Organization. (2009). Medical eligibility criteria for contraceptive use. A WHO family planning cornerstone. WHO Library Cataloguing-in-Publication Data, 4th edition. Geneva: World Health Organization; 2009.

20
CHAPTER

Preconception Care

Usha Sriram

INTRODUCTION

Women of today are at greater risk for noncommunicable diseases and other health issues at a young age. Urbanization and globalization and changing profile of the woman who wishes to get pregnant have added many layers of complexity to women's health status. Sedentary lifestyle, unhealthy eating habits, stress, and older age at pregnancy are some of the reasons why women are predisposed to poor pregnancy outcomes (Fig. 1).

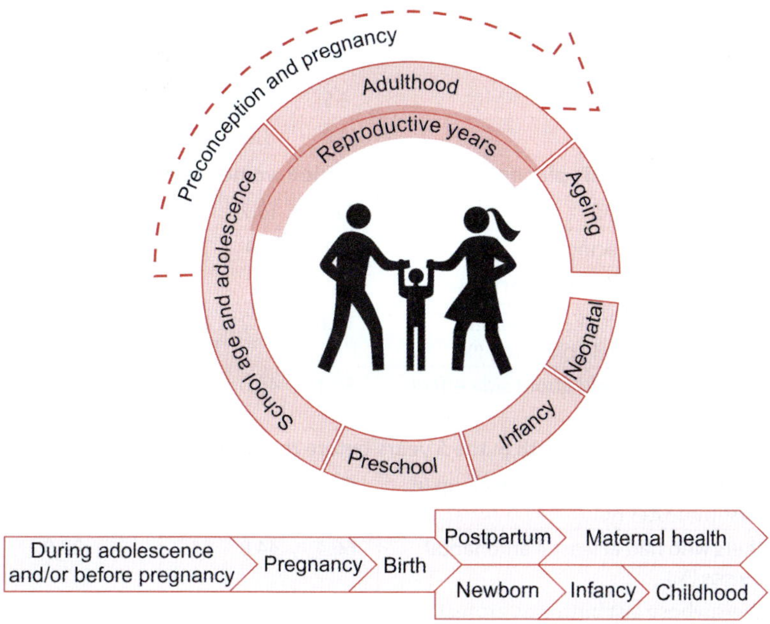

FIG. 1 Lifestyle and preconception care

The World Health Organization defines preconception care as the provision of biomedical, behavioral, and social health interventions to women and couples before conception occurs. It aims at improving their health status, and reducing behaviors and individual and environmental factors that contribute to poor maternal and child health outcomes.

RATIONALE FOR PRECONCEPTION CARE

The four compelling reasons for preconception care are:

1. As many as 40% of all pregnancies are unplanned (globally) and more than 50% of women in India do not use any form of birth control. The latest National Family Health Survey data is presented in table 1.

Table 1: Data of the latest National Family Health Survey

Indicators	NFHS-4 (2015-16)			NFHS-3 (2005-06)
Population and household profile	**Urban**	**Rural**	**Total**	**Total**
Infant and child mortality rates (per 1,000 live birth)				
Infant mortality rate	29	46	41	57
Under-five mortality rate	34	56	50	74
Current use of family planning methods (currently married women age 15–49 years)				
Any method (%)	57.2	51.7	53.5	56.3
Any modern method (%)	51.3	46.0	47.8	48.5
Female sterilization (%)	35.7	36.1	36.0	37.3
Male sterilization (%)	0.3	0.3	0.3	1.0
IUD/PPIUD (%)	2.4	1.1	1.5	1.7
Pill (%)	3.5	4.3	4.1	3.1
Condom (%)	9.0	3.9	5.6	5.2
Unmet need for family planning (currently married women age 15–49 years)				
Total unmet need (%)	12.1	13.2	12.9	13.9
Unmet need for spacing (%)	5.1	5.9	5.7	6.1
Quality of family planning services				
Health worker ever talked to female nonusers about family planning (%)	18.6	17.2	17.7	10.1
Current users ever told about side effects of current method (%)	50.1	45.0	46.5	34.4
Maternity care (for last birth in the 5 years before the survey)				
Mothers who had antenatal check-up in the first trimester (%)	69.1	54.2	58.6	43.9
Mothers who had at least 4 antenantal care visits (%)	66.4	44.8	51.2	37.0
Mothers whose last birth was protected against neonatal tetanus (%)	89.9	88.6	89.0	76.3

Continued

Continued

Table 1: Data of the latest National Family Health Survey

Indicators	NFHS-4 (2015-16)			NFHS-3 (2005-06)
Mothers who consumed iron folic acid for 100 days or more when they were pregnant (%)	40.8	25.9	30.3	15.2
Mothers who had full antenantal care (%)	31.1	16.7	21.0	11.6
Registered pregnancies for which the mother received mother and child protection card (%)	87.7	90.0	89.3	NA
Mothers who received postnatal care from a doctor/nurse/LHV/ANM/midwife/other health personnel within 2 days of delivery (%)	71.7	58.5	62.4	34.6
Mothers who received financial assistance under Janani Suraksha Yojana for births delivered in an institution (%)	21.4	43.8	36.4	NA
Average out of pocket expenditure per delivery in public health facility (Rs)	3,913	2,947	3,198	Na
Children born at home who were taken to a health facility for check-up within 24 hours of birth (%)	3.2	2.4	2.5	0.3
Children who received a health check after birth from a doctor/nurse/LHV/ANM/midwife/other health personnel within 2 days of birth (%)	27.2	23.0	24.3	Na
Nutritional status of adults (age 15–49 years)				
Women whose body mass index (BMI) is below normal (BMI <18.5 kg/m^2) (%)	15.5	26.7	22.9	35.5
Men whose body mass index is below normal (BMI <18.5 kg/m^2) (%)	15.3	23.0	20.2	34.2
Women who are overweight or obese (BMI ≥25.0 kg/m^2) (%)	31.3	15.0	20.7	12.6
Men who are overweight or obese (BMI ≥25.0 kg/m^2) (%)	26.3	14.3	18.6	9.3
Anemia among children and adults				
Children age 6–59 months who are anemic (<11.0 g/dL) (%)	55.9	59.4	58.4	69.4
Nonpregnant women age 15–49 years who are anemic (<12.0 g/dL) (%)	50.9	54.3	53.1	55.2
Pregnant women age 15–49 years who are anemic (<11.0 g/dL) (%)	45.7	52.1	50.3	57.9
All women age 15–49 years who are anemic (%)	50.8	54.2	53.0	55.3
Men age 15–49 years who are anemic (<13.0 g/dL) (%)	18.4	25.1	22.7	24.2

IUD, intrauterine devices; PPIUD, postpartum intrauterine devices; LVH,lady health visitor; ANM, auxiliary nurse midwife.

2. The first 6–10 weeks are critical for organogenesis and many women may seek antenatal care only after this period or towards the end of this critical period.
3. Many preventable and treatable conditions can be easily identified by a simple clinical evaluation by simple history taking critical risks like smoking, tobacco use, alcohol, drug use, medication history, stress, domestic violence, physical activity, environmental exposure etc. can be assessed.
4. Maternal mortality is still unacceptably high in some countries. Anemia is a common treatable condition that contributes significantly to maternal mortality.

BENEFITS OF PRECONCEPTION CARE

It is now well established that preconception care can prevent majority of pregnancy related complications and improve outcomes. Changing certain behaviors, folic acid intake, optimizing nutrition and body weight, stress reduction, and proactive measures like immunization can go a very long way in terms of having an uncomplicated pregnancy and preventing low birth weight and preterm deliveries. Pregnancy is now considered a "window" to future risk of chronic diseases in the mother as is low birth weight as a risk factor for future diabetes and heart disease in the child (Fig. 1).

Beginning the preconception care program early in a young woman's life will benefit her in many ways even if she is not planning a pregnancy in the immediate future. It begins a culture of healthy eating, physical activity, reduction in risky behavior, and correction of nutritional deficiencies.

Preconception Checklist for All Women Developed by Diabetes in Women Worldwide Awareness Advocacy Action Strategies

- **Anemia:** Common cause of maternal mortality, preterm delivery evaluation, and treatment
- **Alcohol:** Any amount of alcohol drinking during pregnancy increases risk of fetal alcohol syndrome. Alcohol cessation counseling
- **Blood pressure:** Blood pressure check, review of medications, changing to medicines that are safe during pregnancy
- **Body mass index (BMI)/weight:** Overweight and obesity is on the rise among Indian women. Undernutrition is still a significant problem particularly in rural areas. Calculate BMI. Nutritional evaluation and counseling
- **Contraception:** Women need education counseling, and guidance
- **Diabetes:** Pregestational diabetes and gestational diabetes mellitus (GDM) are associated with serious maternal and fetal risks. Screening for glucose intolerance is recommended for all women planning a pregnancy

- **Domestic violence:** Verbal and physical by partner and family can affect women's health during pregnancy and baby's weight. Women need counseling on ill effects
- **Environmental and occupational exposure:** Occupational exposure, cooking fuels, exposure to lead and mercury, and pesticides could lead to birth defects and poor pregnancy outcomes. Detailed history and counseling regarding the potential risks is needed
- **Folic acid:** 0.4 mg of folic acid begun 3 months before pregnancy and continued through first trimester can prevent major neural tube defects
- **Family health history:** Diabetes, hypertension, heart disease, and genetic disorders
- **Health history:** History of medical conditions, surgical history, medication use, and allergies
- **Obstetrics and gynecological history:** Obstetrics and gynecological history of subfertility, prior pregnancy losses, complications, baby weight, polycystic ovary syndrome, pelvic infections, and surgery
- **Immunizations/infections:** Vaccine-preventable diseases like rubella, tetanus and diphtheria, hepatitis B, and chicken pox should be addressed during the preconception period. Counseling regarding certain infections like influenza, zika, and human immunodeficiency virus have to be provided to the mother
- **Medications:** Many medications that includes prescription medications, over the counter medications, herbal supplements, and vitamins
- **Mental health:** Many Indian women may have mental illness like depression, anxiety, and schizophrenia that they may not disclose for fear of being rejected and social isolation
- **Nutrition:** Nutritional deficiencies are common in young women and the dual burden both overweight and underweight exists in our country. A detailed diet history and laboratory assessment when indicated will assist in counseling
- **Physical activity:** A physically inactive woman is likely to have a poor metabolic profile, low vitamin D, more overweight and face the consequences such as gestational diabetes and hypertension. Conversely an active woman will remain active and have less chances of GDM and other complications
- **Partner/spousal health:** The partner's health is also vital in the whole preconception care scheme
- **Recreational drugs:** Drugs such as marijuana, cocaine, methamphetamine, and other drugs are implicated in maternal health problems due to addiction, fetal health problems due to illicit drugs used, and low birth weight. Deaddiction programs have to be recommended
- **Sexually transmitted infections:** Gonorrhea, chlamydia, hepatitis, syphilis, and other sexually transmitted infections can lead to subfertility and congenital infections

- **Smoking/tobacco:** Smoking has been linked to poor pregnancy outcomes, preterm delivery, and low birth weight. Toxins related to nicotine can cause damage to fetal genetic material. Smoking cessation guidance needs to be provided
- **Stress:** Anxiety, poor sleep, work pressure, and attention deficit are common in young women now. Stress reduction measures will help in improving outcomes
- **Socioeconomic, cultural context:** Preconception care should also be addressed in terms of her education, health literacy, socioeconomic status, and ethnicity and cultural context
- **Thyroid:** Hypothyroidism (overt and subclinical), thyroid autoimmunity are important health issues that need to assessed and thyroid hormone levels optimized
- **Vitamin D:** Low levels of vitamin D have been associated with obesity, metabolic syndrome, osteomalacia, and newborn rickets. Evaluation and appropriate correction (supplements, diet, and sun exposure).

SELECT CLINICAL SITUATIONS

Pregestational Diabetes

Women with type 1 and type 2 diabetes are at much greater risk for pregnancy losses, pregnancy-induced hypertension, intrauterine growth retardation, macrosomia and intrauterine death, and birth defects. Pre-GDM is a brilliant example of remarkable improvements in outcome with planned pregnancy and optimization of glycemic control, medications, comorbidities, and nutrition.

Combined incidence of major malformation and spontaneous abortion according to the glycosylated hemoglobin (HbA1c) value during the first trimester of pregnancy in 303 women with type 1 diabetes mellitus. The risk rose markedly at HbA1c values above 11% (approximately equivalent to an HbA1c value of 8.5%). Other studies have found an increase in risk at HbA1c values above 9.5%.

In addition to routine prenatal assessment, women with pregestational diabetes will need thyroid-stimulating hormone, HbA1c, renal function, eye exam, and cardiac evaluation. Provision of effective contraception while the woman is being evaluated and getting ready for her pregnancy is equally important.

Targeted Preconception Physical Examination for Women with Diabetes

- Dilated funduscopic examination by an ophthalmologist
- Examination for thyromegaly
- Cardiac auscultation
- Evaluation for carotid bruits and pulses present to the periphery

- Blood pressure measurement in both arms and pulse, lying and standing to check for orthostasis
- Lung auscultation
- Check for succession splash if patient not fasting
- Check sensation and check for tremor, hypo- or hyperreflexia.

GESTATIONAL DIABETES

Gestational diabetes has risen to alarming proportions especially in Southeast Asia (International Diabetes Federation atlas 7 indicates that 25% of pregnancies in Southeast Asia could be complicated by hyperglycemia). Modifiable risk factors like preconception weight and physical activity need to be addressed aggressively to decrease the burden in women of child bearing age and diabetes in their offspring. By preconception screening, all women with prediabetes, undiagnosed diabetes, and metabolic syndrome can be identified and preventive measures initiated. All women of Indian origin are at risk for diabetes and especially those with family history, who are overweight, lead a sedentary life, have polycystic ovary syndrome, previous poor pregnancy outcome, and those born low birth weight.

Young women are increasingly being diagnosed with prediabetes and overt type 2 diabetes mellitus as shown in this study from India are likely to develop GDM if appropriate nutritional changes and activity are not made.

While GDM is a diagnosis that is not made before conception, attempts to prevent GDM can be made with preconception screening of blood glucose.

SCREENING FOR GENETIC CONDITIONS (WORLD HEALTH ORGANIZATION RECOMMENDATIONS)

- Screening for anemia
- Taking a thorough family history
- Family planning
- Genetic counseling
- Carrier screening and testing
- Appropriate treatment
- Providing community-based education
- Community-wide or national screening among populations at high risk
- Population-wide screening.

PROVIDING GUIDANCE AND INFORMATION ON ENVIRONMENTAL HAZARDS AND PREVENTION (WORLD HEALTH ORGANIZATION RECOMMENDATIONS)

- Protecting from unnecessary radiation exposure in occupational, environmental, and medical settings

- Avoiding unnecessary pesticide use/providing alternatives to pesticides
- Protecting from lead exposure
- Informing women of childbearing age about levels of methylmercury in fish
- Promoting use of improved stoves and cleaner liquid/gaseous fuels.

SEXUALLY TRANSMITTED INFECTIONS (WORLD HEALTH ORGANIZATION RECOMMENDATIONS)

- Providing age-appropriate comprehensive sexuality education and services
- Promoting safe sex practices through individual, group, and community-level behavioral interventions
- Promoting condom use for dual protection against sexually transmitted infections and unwanted pregnancies
- Ensuring increased access to condoms
- Screening for sexually transmitted infections
- Increasing access to treatment and other relevant health services.

CONCLUSION

With dedicated program that will ensure that all women are screened, counseled, and given directions, many pregnancy related complications and maternal mortality will decrease and a healthy baby with optimum weight and without birth defects can be a reality.

Focus on maternal mortality and women's reproductive health has been extremely successful. With preconception care, proper and timely antenatal care, and postpartum follow up, the goal of reaching less than 100 maternal deaths/100,000 pregnancies will become a reality.

All healthcare providers, community health workers, advocacy groups, and policy makers, and, in short, a multisectoral approach will be needed to participate in this effort to make it successful.

SUGGESTED READINGS

1. American College of Obstetricians and Gynecologists Committee on Health Care for Undeserved Women. ACOG Committee Opinion No. 343: psychosocial risk factors: perinatal screening and intervention. Obstet Gynecol. 2006;108(2):469-77.
2. Centers for Disease Control and Prevention. Preconception health and healthcare. Avaiable from: www.cdc.gov/preconception/index.html.
3. Dunlop AL, Jack B, Frey K. National recommendations for preconception care: The essential role of the family physician. J Am Board Fam Med. 2007;20(1):81-4.
4. Good clinical practice recommendations on preconception care. Available from: http://www.fogsi.org/gcpr-preconception-care/.

5. NFHS4 National Family health Survey India. Available from: http://rchiips.org/NFHS/factsheet_NFHS-4.shtml.
6. Poels M, Koski MP, Boejie HR, et al. Why do women not use preconception care? A systematic review on barriers and facilitators. Obstet Gynecol Surv. 2016;71(10):603-12.
7. Preconception care: Maximizing the gain for maternal and child health. Available from: www.who.int/maternal_child_adolescent/document/preconceptioncare_policy-brief
8. Preconception care and prenatal care: Overview-NICHD. Available from: www.nichd.nih.gov/health/topics/preconceptioncare/pages/default.aspe.
9. Vaccination for women FOGSI. Available from: http://www.fogsi.org/wp-content/uploads/2015/11/vaccination_women.pdf

21

CHAPTER

Breastfeeding and Diabetes

Viveka P Jyotsna, Nishant Raizada

INTRODUCTION

Breastfeeding is an important physiological event in the postpartum period. While on one hand breastfeeding reduces childhood morbidity and mortality, on the other hand multiple health benefits accrue to the mother as well. With the rising prevalence of prediabetes and diabetes, the number of pregnancies complicated by gestational or pregestational diabetes is also increasing. The effect of breastfeeding on future diabetes risk and problems in breastfeeding in pregnancies complicated by diabetes is an interesting as well as important topic.

BREASTFEEDING PREVALENCE IN DIABETES

Data from a large cohort in the United States showed that prevalence of breastfeeding initiation (BFI) in women with gestational diabetes mellitus (GDM) and pregestational diabetes were 80.2 and 78.2%, respectively. The BFI rates in pregestational diabetes were significantly lower than that in nondiabetic mothers (82.2%). The breastfeeding continuation rates were 65.7% in GDM and 60.4% in pregestational diabetes; both were significantly lesser than nondiabetic mothers (68.8%).While other studies also report similar BFI rates in GDM and nondiabetic mothers, women with GDM tended to initiate introduction of formula feeds within 2 days of birth.

Women with GDM have lower rates of breastfeeding at discharge and lower predominant breastfeeding rates as compared to women without diabetes. Women with type 2 diabetes mellitus (T2DM) were less likely to breastfeed as the first feed compared to GDM women and were also less likely to be breastfeeding at discharge. A systematic review also found that a delayed onset of lactation was associated with diabetes in pregnancy (DIP).

Women with type 1 diabetes mellitus (T1DM) have breastfeeding rates at birth comparable to those with T2DM and were more likely to be breastfeeding at 4 months postpartum compared to T2DM women.

In India, early (within 1 hour of delivery) breastfeeding was seen in 40.5% and exclusive breastfeeding was found in 54.6% in the general population. Data on breastfeeding in mothers with gestational or pregestational diabetes in India are not available.

FACTORS AFFECTING BREASTFEEDING AND BREASTFEEDING BEHAVIOR IN DIABETES

Prepregnancy obesity was associated with lower rates of breastfeeding at discharge and at 4 months postpartum in both T2DM and GDM. Even in euglycemic women, higher BMI impairs lactation. Further maternal fat distribution in additional to BMI plays a part, with more abdominal fat associated with lower probability of breastfeeding.

Insulin resistance is another factor contributing to abnormalities in breastfeeding. Insulin plays a role in lactation including differentiation and activation of secretory cells and mature milk production. Insulin-sensitive gene expression has been found to be upregulated during lactation. It is postulated that insulin resistance interferes with these processes. Early cessation of exclusive breastfeeding was more common in women with abnormal 1 hour glucose challenge test compared to those with normal glucose challenge tests. Insulin treatment is also associated with delayed lactogenesis in GDM women. Poor glycemic control in GDM and T2DM is also associated with delayed onset of lactation—insulin resistance is the underlying factor in both these disorders. Further supporting this hypothesis, a study found that in T1DM mothers, likelihood of breastfeeding at 2 months postpartum did not depend on HbA1c, duration of diabetes or prepregnancy insulin dose. Maternal education and breastfeeding at discharge were the only significant predictors of likelihood of breastfeeding at 2 months in this study. Thus, poor glycemic control and insulin treatment may just be indicators of severity of insulin resistance rather than independent factors. Breastfeeding as the first feed appears to be a major predictor of breastfeeding at discharge in T2DM and GDM.

However, women with insulin dependent diabetes mellitus did experience delayed lactogenesis in one study as indicated by lower lactose and higher total nitrogen concentrations in breast milk at 2–3 days postpartum. Milk immunoreactive prolactin is lower in T1DM and milk lactose levels increased late in T1DM compared to mothers without diabetes.

Babies born to mothers with diabetes requiring insulin therapy had immature suckling patterns (lesser sucks per burst and lesser bursts) compared to diabetic mothers not needing insulin as well as nondiabetic mothers. This may indicate some neurological immaturity in these newborns.

Lack of education about breastfeeding, inadequate support, more frequent surgical procedures, nipple abnormalities and infections are some other factors which could be operational in women with diabetes.

BREASTFEEDING AND FUTURE DIABETES IN THE MOTHER

There are data to suggest that breastfeeding in nondiabetic mothers can reduce the future risk of T2DM by 32%. Longer periods of breastfeeding were associated by greater reduction in risk of future type 2 diabetes.

Breastfeeding has been shown to have improved glycemic parameters in women with GDM. In women with GDM, breastfeeding during the 2-hour 75 g oral glucose tolerance test (OGTT) was found to reduce plasma 2-hour glucose and insulin concentrations. In the Study of Women, Infant Feeding, and T2DM (SWIFT) cohort of GDM patients, at 6–9 weeks postpartum, exclusive or mostly breastfeeding group had with lower prevalence of prediabetes and diabetes compared to exclusive or mostly formula feeding group. Similarly, in the Atlantic DIP study, dysglycemia at 12 weeks postpartum in GDM was significantly lower in those who had breastfed. At 4 years after delivery, GDM women who lactated had lower fasting and post OGTT (2 hours) blood insulin along with lesser area under the curve for insulin. Higher values on homeostatic model assessment for insulin sensitivity and Matsuda indices were also seen in those who had lactated.

Several studies have shown a decreased incidence of T2DM in GDM mothers who had breastfed. Breastfeeding initiation was associated with an 18–22% reduction in risk of T2DM over 24 years of follow-up in a study from Canada. Further, increasing duration of breastfeeding was associated with lower risk of future diabetes. The median time to diabetes onset after GDM in a German cohort was 12.3 years in women who had breastfed compared with 2.3 years in women who did not breastfeed. However, a recent meta-analysis found that absence of breastfeeding was not associated with increased risk of future risk of T2DM in women with GDM.

In women with T1DM, breastfeeding was associated with lesser glycemic variability without causing hypoglycemia. The total daily dose of insulin decreases during lactation in T1DM by about 13%.

Breastfeeding is associated with increased insulin-mediated glucose uptake which contributes to reduction in hyperinsulinemia and promotes lipid and triglyceride utilization. Lower leptin and visfatin levels with breastfeeding have also been reported.

BENEFITS FOR THE CHILD

Babies born to mothers with GDM when breastfed in the delivery room had significantly lower rates of hypoglycemia and had higher fasting plasma glucose compared to those not breastfed in delivery room.

Breastfeeding for more than 6 months in women with GDM was associated with decreased risk of childhood obesity at 2 years of age. Gestational diabetes mellitus offspring who were breastfed more than 12 months has a 72% reduction in obesity prevalence at 2–4 years of age as compared to GDM offspring who were not breastfed. Slower body mass index (BMI) growth trajectory, lower waist circumference, and subcutaneous and visceral fat was seen in children (born out of pregnancies complicated with diabetes) who were breastfed more than 6 months compared to those breastfed less than 6 months.

In the Pima Indians, pregnancies affected by GDM resulted in lower diabetes prevalence in the offspring who were breastfed (30.1%) compared to those bottle fed (43.6%). Exclusive breastfeeding in first 2 months of life was associated with lower risk of T2DM in Pima Indians aged 10–39 years. Breastfeeding initiation was associated with a 17% reduction in youth onset T2DM in the offspring. Breastfeeding of any duration was associated with lesser risk of developing T2DM with greater reductions with increasing duration of breastfeeding.

PUTATIVE ADVERSE EFFECTS OF BREASTFEEDING

The volume of diabetic breast milk consumed in first week of life has been correlated with risk of overweight at 2 years of age as well as with delay in onset of speaking. However, the sample size was small and subsequent research does not support these observations.

INDIAN DATA

Indian data are scanty. A study from India has looked at impact of breastfeeding and glucose intolerance in late childhood. Longer duration of breastfeeding was associated with lesser risk of glucose intolerance at 9.5 years of age. The children with more than 5 years of breastfeeding had lower homeostasis model assessment for insulin resistance as well.

ORAL HYPOGLYCEMIC AGENTS DURING BREASTFEEDING

Metformin is secreted into breast milk with concentrations varying from 0.25–1.0% of maternal weight adjusted dose. A prospective study of polycystic ovary syndrome mothers taking metformin during pregnancy as well as lactation has not reported any adverse effects on the offspring. Glyburide and glipizide were not detected in breast milk at 5–10 mg doses and the breastfed infants did not show any hypoglycemia in a small study.

PROMOTING BREASTFEEDING IN DIABETIC WOMEN

Maternal education about breastfeeding appears to be the single most important factor which can improve breastfeeding rates. In a study on GDM women, a tailored breastfeeding education and support program implemented starting 22–36 weeks of pregnancy resulted in significantly lesser risk of discontinuing breastfeeding in early as well as late postpartum period. Maternal nutrition therapy in GDM women also increases chances of exclusive breastfeeding at 4 months after delivery.

The effect of breastfeeding education on T2DM education is anticipated although not yet supported by evidence. Additionally, ensuring good metabolic control in women with T2DM is also effective in increasing chances of breastfeeding initiation and continuation.

Facilitation of early breastfeeding (or milk expression) in early postpartum period is needed to prevent delayed BFI and support should be given to reduce perceived delay in second stage of lactogenesis. Antenatal breast milk expression is not recommended in light of available data.

In a recent literature review, the authors noted that concerns regarding breastfeeding (rather than diabetes per se) are the major cause of cessation of breastfeeding. Hence, addressing these concerns through education is the most important step that should be taken to promote breastfeeding. Antenatal counseling regarding benefits of breastfeeding should be started and doubts or myths should be addressed. Local factors such as nipple abnormalities and skin infections should be taken care of. Attempts should be made to ensure BFI as early as feasible but at least within 60 minutes of a vaginal delivery. Rooming in should be promoted and exclusive breastfeeding should be the target in the initial 6 months of life.

To summarize, breastfeeding in diabetic women is associated with a reduction in risk of future obesity and T2DM in the child with possibly reduced risk of progression to T2DM in the mother. Breastfeeding rates in diabetes can be improved by education and promotion of breastfeeding although glycemic control may also play a role.

SUGGESTED READINGS

1. Fallon A, Dunne F. Breastfeeding practices that support women with diabetes to breastfeed. Diabetes Res Clin Pract. 2015;110(1):10-7.
2. Gunderson EP, Hedderson MM, Chiang V, et al. Lactation intensity and postpartum maternal glucose tolerance and insulin resistance in women with recent GDM: the SWIFT cohort. Diabetes Care. 2012;35(1):50-6.
3. Jäger S, Jacobs S, Kröger J, et al. Breast-feeding and maternal risk of type 2 diabetes: a prospective study and meta-analysis. Diabetologia. 2014;57(7):1355-65.
4. Rayanagoudar G, Hashi AA, Zamora J, et al. Quantification of the type 2 diabetes risk in women with gestational diabetes: a systematic review and meta-analysis of 95,750 women. Diabetologia. 2016;59(7):1403-11.

22
CHAPTER

Menopause and Diabetes Including Hormone Replacement Therapy

Surya K Singh, Shweta Bhandari, Balram Gupta

INTRODUCTION

Diabetes mellitus is the most common chronic disease after the age of 30 years with rising prevalence in the advancing age. Consequently, chance of developing type 2 diabetes mellitus (T2DM) is higher in the menopausal females. Both of these are main predisposing factors for cardiovascular disease, a leading cause of death in women in Western world as well as in India. We discussed the relationship between diabetes mellitus in menopausal women with reference to hormone replacement therapy (HRT).

MENOPAUSE IN WOMEN WITH DIABETES

During the time of menopause, women experience vasomotor symptoms, vaginal dryness, and urinary incontinence very frequently. Whether these symptoms are different in women with and without diabetes mellitus was never investigated. Women with diabetes mellitus might have difficulty in differentiating vasomotor symptoms from hypoglycemia. This could lead to increase in dietary intake in response to what are thought to be hypoglycemic symptoms but are in fact vasomotor symptoms. Such perception causes increased food intake leading to hyperglycemia and weight gain over period of time. On the contrary, they can put themselves at risk of drug induced hypoglycemia if they are not able to identify true hypoglycemia for vasomotor symptoms during course of treatment of diabetes mellitus.

Diabetes can increase the reproductive aging and lead to premature ovarian failure or early menopause by various mechanisms. Studies have shown that women with type 1 diabetes mellitus (T1DM) or T2DM have menopause earlier than nondiabetic women. In another study, no difference was found. In T1DM, it might be because of its association with premature ovarian failure as a part of type 2 autoimmune polyglandular syndrome.

Literature is scant on hormonal changes occurring in menopause among women with or without diabetes mellitus. Higher free testosterone levels were seen in postmenopausal women with T2DM than in those without diabetes mellitus. The increased free testosterone levels observed among women with diabetes mellitus might be due to decrease in sex-hormone-binding globulin levels due to hyperinsulinemia.

METABOLIC EFFECTS OF MENOPAUSE

Effects of Menopause on Body Composition and Energy Balance

In females, it is difficult to separate the cellular effects of the normal aging process on body composition from those of menopause. Cross-sectional and longitudinal studies have shown increased fat mass, increased abdominal fat and decreased lean body mass. The cause of the increased abdominal fat has been suggested to be secondary to decreased basal metabolic rate without change in food intake. Both increased visceral fat and decreased lean mass contribute to impair insulin sensitivity. These changes in body composition causing insulin resistance are risk factors predisposing to T2DM after menopause independent of E2 deficiency.

Study by Sowers et al. showed that changes in the level of follicle-stimulating hormone were associated with changes in fat mass, waist circumference, and lean body mass over time, independent of age, which suggested that ovarian aging could be directly linked with menopause-associated changes in body composition.

Insulin Sensitivity

Relationship between abdominal obesity and insulin resistance is well known and it is true in postmenopausal women also. However, several studies failed to show association between menopausal status and homeostatic model assessment measurements of insulin resistance (HOMA-IR).

In the Postmenopausal Estrogen-Progestin Interventions (PEPI) study, a secondary analysis of data on women who were not taking estrogen showed an independent association between increased body mass index (BMI) and waist-to-hip ratio with increased fasting and postchallenge levels of glucose and insulin.

Effect of Menopause on Glucose Homeostasis and Diabetes

Whether menopause affects diabetes risk or not remains controversial. Study done by Soriguer et al. found no association between menopausal status and the prevalence of T2DM. The Study of Women across the Nation

(SWAN) reported an increased incidence of the metabolic syndrome among perimenopausal women, such that by the time the women reached menopause, 13.7% of the study group had developed this syndrome. Increased levels of free testosterone have been associated with an increased risk of impaired fasting glucose and T2DM in postmenopausal women. In the SWAN study, the incidence of the metabolic syndrome was increased in women with high levels of bioavailable testosterone or low levels of sex-hormone-binding globulin. In a recent prospective cohort study from the Women's Health Initiative (WHI), it was found that total endogenous estrogen exposure (difference between age of menarche and final menstrual period) also predisposed to the risk of T2DM. Women with smallest (<30 year) reproductive time had a 37% increased risk of developing T2DM, while women with the greater (45+ year) reproductive time had a 23% more risk than women with medium-length reproductive periods (36–40 year). Consequently, the preponderance of facts argues for a role of menopausal E2 deficiency in the increased risk of T2DM. On the other hand, an increased cumulative of E2 exposure may also predispose to T2DM.

Effects of Menopause on Complications of Diabetes

Urinary incontinence is very much prevalent among postmenopausal women. Mechanisms by which diabetes causes incontinence are:

- Microvascular injury to the innervations of the bladder and urethral sphincter
- Detrusor muscle and sphincter dysfunction
- Urinary retention and increased postvoid residual urine leading to overflow incontinence, chronic bacterial overgrowth, and urinary tract infection
- Uncontrolled blood glucose levels.

On the contrary, a study fails to demonstrate any difference in urinary incontinence in postmenopausal women with or without diabetes mellitus. Even though diabetes mellitus is associated with greater severity of incontinence, this could be due to differences in BMI between women with diabetes mellitus compared to those without diabetes.

POSTMENOPAUSAL HORMONE THERAPY

Mechanisms of postmenopausal hormone therapy are discussed below.

Antidiabetic Actions

The incidence of T2DM may be slightly lower in postmenopausal HRT users than nonusers. Several studies have examined the effect of hormone therapy on diabetes risk in postmenopausal women. In secondary analysis of Heart and Estrogen-Progestin Replacement Study (HERS), combined conjugated equine estrogen and medroxyprogesterone acetate (MPA) was associated with a 35% reduction in the incidence diabetes mellitus as compared to women who received placebo. The absolute reduction in diabetes mellitus incidence in the women who received hormone therapy was 3.3% over the 4.1 years of follow-up, or 0.8% fewer cases per year than in the group that received placebo.

Similarly, in a secondary analysis of the WHI hormone trial, the cumulative incidence of T2DM was 3.5% among women who received hormone therapy, whereas it was 4.2% among women who received placebo.

However, in the HERS and WHI trials, the diabetes prevention observed in women assigned to menopausal hormonal therapy (MHT) was independent from the observed reduction in BMI and waist circumference. Therefore, available evidence suggests that estrogens improve glucose homeostasis via acting directly on estrogen receptor (ER) stress in liver and skeletal muscle (or adipose tissue) to improve insulin sensitivity, or on ER stress in pancreatic islets to improve insulin secretion, as can be observed in rodent models. Thus, the antidiabetic effect of MHT may involve mechanisms that are similar or different than those of endogenous E2 and are not necessarily mirroring the defects observed during menopause.

COMPARISON OF ORAL AND TRANSDERMAL ESTROGEN DELIVERY

As compared to orally administered estrogens, transdermal E2 delivery avoids first pass liver metabolism, leading to more stable systemic E2 levels without supraphysiological liver exposure to estrogens and higher systemic E2 levels. Thus, transdermal E2 provides more physiological delivery of hormone into the circulation without the side effects of oral conjugated estrogens (CE) therapy on hepatic synthesis of triglycerides, clotting factors, and inflammatory markers. However, oral CE causes greater reduction in low density lipoprotein (LDL)/high density lipoprotein (HDL) ratio, higher beneficial effect on insulin resistance (HOMA-IR) leading to a better suppression of hepatic glucose production because of first pass liver metabolism. In short, both oral and transdermal E2 can lower blood glucose and improve insulin sensitivity with oral CE having the more powerful effect at equivalent doses.

EFFECT OF PROGESTOGENS ON GLUCOSE AND INSULIN MET ABOLISM

The type of progestogen used in combined therapy influences the effect on insulin sensitivity. Medroxyprogesterone acetate, and similarly levonogesterol, results in a deterioration of insulin resistance. Nonandrogenic progestogens norethisterone have a neutral effect. Dydrogesterone shows a neutral effect when added to CE. Thus, MPA and levonorgestrel are more likely to be associated with attenuation of the beneficial effect of estrogen on glucose homeostasis, while norethisterone acetate and dydrogesterone are more likely to be neutral. With most progestogens, the reversal of the beneficial effect of E2 or CE is dose- dependent.

Diabetes, Hormone Replacement Therapy, and Lipid Metabolism

The WHI trial demonstrated that HRT decreases LDL-C (–12.7%), and increase HDL-C (7.3%) and triglycerides (6.9%) levels. These findings are similar with those with HERS and PEPI studies. Low-dose HRT seems to be superior to conventional HRT. Although, oral conjugated equine estrogen therapy only could lead to high levels of triglycerides (25%) and increases the risk of pancreatitis.

Cardiovascular Disease and Diabetes

Coronary Heart Disease

The HERS trial found that 4.1 years of daily combined therapy in postmenopausal women with coronary heart disease (CHD) did not decrease overall CHD risk. Various explanations have been given for the overall null and void effect of HRT in HERS, which included the dual effect of estrogen (early risk and late benefit) and the age of the women (mean age was 66.7 years).

Data on the effects of HRT on CHD are inconsistent and a major factor is timing. The WHI studies established that women who were started hormone therapy nearer to the menopause tended to have a decreased CHD risk compared with the higher risk among women who were started HRT later. As a result, HRT might be helpful in younger (<60 years) postmenopausal diabetic women, but it cannot be recommended exclusively for the prevention of cardiovascular disease. Therefore, it should not be prescribed for older diabetic women with additional cardiovascular risk factors.

Stroke

Stroke is more prevalent in diabetics. Postmenopausal HRT is a well-documented, independent, and modifiable risk factor for stroke. Both HRT arms of the WHI study found an increase in ischemic stroke.

Venous Thromboembolism

Both diabetes and oral HRT are associated with increased risk of (venous thromboembolism) VTE. Transdermal HRT may be associated with a lower risk. Also type of progestogens also influence the risk, norpregnane derivative may have higher thrombogenic risk as compared to micronized progesterone and pregnane derivatives which do not increase risk.

Cancer and Diabetes

Diabetes is an independent risk factor for development of endometrial cancer. Obese women, women with high BMI, are at higher risk due to increased levels of estrogen. High prevalence of T2DM in obese people indicates this common etiology of both conditions. If uterus is present it is necessary that they are given progestogen to prevent endometrial carcinoma.

There is a possible link between diabetes and breast cancer but no strong evidence is available for postmenopausal diabetic HRT users. The 2008 EMAS consensus statement concluded that the risk in breast cancer increases with duration of treatment and is more with estrogen-progestogen compared to estrogen-only therapy.

The incidence of colorectal cancer is higher in T2DM patients. In WHI study, HRT reduces the risk of colorectal cancer; little is known about colorectal cancer risk when treatment is stopped.

Principles of Management of Diabetic Women at the Menopause

In young T2DM women (50–59 years of age and within 10 years after menopause), MHT improves glycemic control, with oral estrogens providing a stronger improvement in insulin sensitivity than transdermal E2 at equivalent doses.

Therefore, in normal weight diabetic women, an oral route of estrogen delivery may be preferred only if the 10-year atherosclerotic cardiovascular disease (ASCVD) risk is low. Oral estrogens have beneficial effects on HDL and LDL cholesterol and may be prescribed in normal weight women with T2DM, because they produce a greater improvement in insulin sensitivity.

In diabetic women with a moderate 10-year risk of ASCVD or/and in obese diabetic women, transdermal E2 will be favored along with a progesterone which is neutral on coagulation and insulin sensitivity. Transdermal E2 has more positive effects on inflammatory markers and triglycerides than CE does and may not increase risk of VTE.

Finally, in elderly women (60 years or more than 10 years after menopause), MHT should initiated on an individual basis and after careful consideration of other risk factors.

CONCLUSION

Diabetes is a major risk factor for cardiovascular disease and the risk is further increased in women with menopause. Managing menopausal women with diabetes is a clinical challenge. Many times symptoms of estrogen deficiency masquerade hypoglycemia and vice versa posing uncertainty of dose modification of antihyperglycemic agents in menopausal women.

Use of HRT needs to be carefully and individually assessed with special consideration to type and route of administration. Nonestrogen-based treatments for menopausal symptoms and osteoporosis is an area that should be developed further.

SUGGESTED READINGS

1. Department of Health. Series DH2. No. 30. Mortality statistics cause review of the registrar general on deaths by cause, sex and age, in England and Wales. London; 2003.
2. Nelson HD. Menopause. Lancet. 2008;371:760-70.
3. Dougherty P, Pastors JG. Women & diabetes. Menopause. What to expect, how to cope. Diabetes Self Manga. 2007;24:84-7.
4. Dorman JS, Steenkiste AR, Foley TP, et al. Menopause in type 1 diabetic women: is it premature? Diabetes. 2001;50:1857-62.
5. Strotmeyer ES, Steenkiste AR, Foley TP Jr, et al. Menstrual cycle differences between women with type 1 diabetes and women without diabetes. Diabetes Care. 2003;26:1016-21.
6. Malacara JM, Huerta R, Rivera B, et al. Menopause in normal and uncomplicated NIDDM women: physical and emotional symptoms and hormone profile. Maturitas. 1997;28:35-45.
7. López-López R, Huerta R, Malacara JM. Age at menopause in women with type 2 diabetes mellitus. Menopause. 1999;6(2):174-8.
8. Eisenbarth, GS, Gottlieb PA. Autoimmune polyendocrine syndromes. N Engl J Med. 2004;350:2068-79.
9. Korytkowski MT, Krug EI, Daly MA, et al. Does androgen excess contribute to the cardiovascular risk profile in postmenopausal women with type 2 diabetes? Metabolism. 2005;54:1626-31.
10. Carr MC. The emergence of the metabolic syndrome with menopause. J Clin Endocrinol Metab. 2003;88:2404-11.
11. Guo SS, Zeller C, Chumlea WC, et al. Aging, body composition, and lifestyle: the FELS longitudinal study. Am J Clin Nutr. 1999;70:405-11.
12. Ley CJ, Lees B, Stevenson JC. Sex- and menopause-associated changes in body-fat distribution. Am J Clin Nutr. 1992;55:950-4.
13. Panotopoulos G, Ruiz JC, Raison J, et al. Menopause, fat and lean distribution in obese women. Maturitas. 1996;25:11-19.
14. Sowers M, Zheng H, Tomey K, et al. Changes in body composition in women over six years at midlife: Ovarian and chronological aging. J Clin Endocrinol Metab. 2007;92:895-901.
15. Sternfeld B, Bhat AK, Wang H, et al. Menopause, physical activity, and body composition/fat distribution in midlife women. Med Sci Sports Exerc. 2005;37:1195-202.
16. Svendsen OL, Hassager C, Christiansen C. Age- and menopause-associated variations in body composition and fat distribution in healthy women as measured by dual-energy X-ray absorptiometry. Metabolism. 1995;44:369-73.
17. Muscelli E, Kozàkovà M, Flyvbjerg A, et al. The effect of menopause on carotid artery remodeling, insulin sensitivity, and plasma adiponectin in healthy women. Am J Hypertens. 2009;4:364-70.
18. Barrett-Connor E, Schrott HG, Greendale G, et al. Factors associated with glucose and insulin levels in healthy postmenopausal women. Diabetes Care. 1996;19:333-40.
19. Soriguer F, Morcillo S, Hernando V, et al. Type 2 diabetes mellitus and other cardiovascular risk factors are no more common during menopause: Longitudinal study. Menopause. 2009;16:817-21.

20. Janssen I, Powell LH, Crasford S, et al. Menopause and the metabolic syndrome: the study of women's health across the nation. Arch Intern Med. 2008;168:1568-75.
21. Golden SH, Dobs AS, Vaidya D, et al. Endogenous sex hormones and glucose tolerance status in postmenopausal women. J Clin Endocrinol Metab. 2007;92:1289-95.
22. Oh JY, Barrett-Connor E, Wedick NM, et al. Endogenous sex hormones and the development of type 2 diabetes in older men and women: the Rancho Bernardo study. Diabetes Care. 2002;25:55-60.
23. Jackson SL, Scholes D, Boyko EJ, et al. Urinary incontinence and diabetes in postmenopausal women. Diabetes Care. 2005;28:1730-8.
24. Kanaya AM, Herrington D, Vittinghoff E, et al. Glycemic effects of postmenopausal hormone therapy: the Heart and Estrogen/Progestin Replacement Study. A randomized, double-blind, placebo-controlled trial. Ann Intern Med. 2003;138:1-9.
25. Margolis KL, Bonds DE, Rodabough RJ, et al. Effect of oestrogen plus progestin on the incidence of diabetes in postmenopausal women: Results from the Women's Health Initiative hormone trial. Diabetologia. 2004;47:1175-87.
26. Godsland IF, Manassiev NA, Felton CV, et al. Effects of low and high dose oestradiol and dydrogesterone therapy on insulin and lipoprotein metabolism in healthy postmenopausal women. Clin Endocrinlol. 2004;60:541-9.
27. Lindheim SR, Presser SC, Ditkoff EC, et al. A possible bimodal effect of strong insulin sensitivity in postmenopausal women and the attenuating effect of added progestin. Fertil Steril. 1993;60:664-7.
28. Luotola H, Pyorala T, Loikkanen M. Effects of natural oestrogen/progestogen substitution therapy on carbohydrate and lipid metabolism in postmenopausal women. Maturitas. 1986;8:245-53.
29. Petitti DB. Hormone replacement therapy and heart disease prevention: experimentation trumps observation. JAMA. 1998;280:650-2.
30. Mosca L, Collins P, Herrington DM, et al. AHA scientific statement: hormone replacement therapy and cardiovascular disease—a statement for healthcare professionals from the American heart association. Circulation. 2001;104:499.
31. Rossouw JE, Prentice RL, Manson JE, et al. Postmenopausal hormone therapy and risk of cardiovascular disease by age and years since menopause. JAMA. 2007;297:1465-77.
32. Tsai AW, Cushman M, Rosamond WD, et al. Cardiovascular risk factors and venous thromboembolism incidence: The longitudinal investigation of thromboembolism aetiology. Arch Intern Med. 2002;162:1182-9.
33. Canonico M, Plu-Bureau G, Lowe GD, et al. Hormone replacement therapy and risk of venous thromboembolism in postmenopausal women: systematic review and meta-analysis. BMJ. 2008;336:1227-31.
34. Rees M, Stevenson J, Hope S, et al. Management of the menopause. 5th ed. London: British Menopause Society Publications Ltd. and Royal Society of Medicine Press; 2009.
35. Nilsen TI, Vatten LJ. Prospective study of colorectal cancer risk and physical activity, diabetes, hyperinsulinemia hypothesis. Br J Cancer. 2001;84:417-22.

23
CHAPTER

Malignancies

Sudha Vidyasagar, Banshi Saboo, Anshul Singh

INTRODUCTION AND EPIDEMIOLOGY

Diabetes and cancer are noncommunicable diseases which are on the rise in today's world. Both these diseases contribute to increasing mortality, morbidity, and economic costs in the form of hospitalization and drug therapy.

In absence of a national registry that would have provided comprehensive cancer incidence or mortality data for India, the current magnitude of the problem at best is an educated guess. The best estimates are as per the International Agency for Research on Cancer GLOBOCAN project, which puts the age-adjusted incidence of cancer as 1,045 per 100,000 among Indian women. This data also reveals that breast cancer and cervical cancer are the most common causes of cancer related deaths in India, both sexes combined. What is more alarming is that the GLOBOCAN estimates these numbers to double over the next 20 years.

INDIAN DATA ON CANCER IN WOMEN WTH DIABETES

In India where both diabetes and cancer are outpacing each other, there are very few studies reporting the same especially in women. The largest numbers are from a case control study undertaken in Kerala which evaluated the role of chronic diseases in the pathogenesis of premalignant oral conditions. A very pertinent result of this study was that diabetes was found to be as an independent risk factor of oral leukoplakia and erythroplakia in women. The odds ratio in this study was found to be more than twofold and it had a statistical significance even after adjustment for potential confounding factors.

A further analysis revealed that the risk was consistently high among women, even in the absence of a history of smoking or consumption of chewable tobacco.

Another study from Pune had looked at the mortality and occurrence of cancer in patients with and without diabetes. They analyzed 14,838 death certificates data for the year 2006, and studied the cases with diabetes and cancer. The data from this study revealed that diabetic females had higher incidence of breast, lung, liver, oral, central nervous system tumors, non-Hodgkin's lymphoma, and laryngeal cancer as compared to nondiabetics. The major drawback of this study was that in a death certificate-based research potentially confounding factors may escape detection hence any association at the best is an assumption.

Diabetes has been increasing to epidemic proportions in India, and the convergence of diabetes and cancer can be disastrous. Women with diabetes form a very vulnerable population as medical care allocated to them socially is always suspect. Cancers of the breast endometrium and ovary which are high in incidence are especially common in diabetic women. In this article, we will try to define the overlap between diabetes and cancer in terms of pathophysiology, presentation, and prognosis.

ASSOCIATION BETWEEN DIABETES AND CANCER

Patients with type 2 diabetes mellitus (T2DM) have a higher incidence of several cancers including carcinoma pancreas, hepatoma, and colonic carcinoma. In addition, women with diabetes have a significantly increased risk of cancers of the breast and endometrium.

PATHOLOGICAL LINK

There are various theories about why cancer is more common among diabetic patients. One of the strong contenders for this association the hyperinsulinemia that occurs in patients with T2DM. Insulin is an anabolic hormone and promotes proliferation. The pancreas, liver, and peripheral organs are exposed to high levels of insulin in patients with T2DM. The binding of insulin to the insulin-like growth factor 1 (IGF-1) receptor may promote antiapoptotic properties of this hormone.

The question then arises about type 1 diabetes mellitus (T1DM) where the insulin levels are actually low or undetectable. However, even in type 1 diabetic patients, breast and endometrial cancers are of a higher incidence. This could be due to the higher incidence of nulliparity and menstrual irregularities in patients with T1DM. However, data on T1DM and cancer is still controversial as a large cohort study from Sweden[6] did not show any clear cut association.

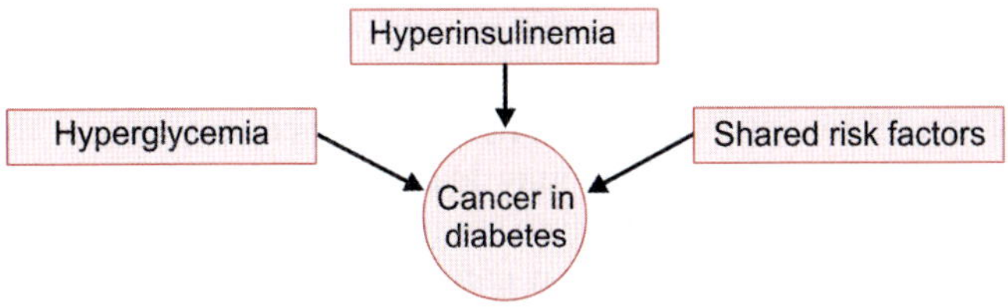

FIG. 1: Pathological link between cancer and diabetes

In addition, the duration of diabetes mellitus may be associated with increasing cancer risk. Whether this is due to patients getting older and cancer being more common in elderly is again unanswered. Further the association of pioglitazone used to treat T2DM causing increased incidence of bladder cancer also complicates the scene.

A second hypothesis postulates that glycemia itself can predispose to cancer. Hyperglycemia may increase vascular proliferation. The Warburg effect proposes that glucose is utilized by cancer cells to proliferate. The ^{18}F-fluorodeoxyglucose-positron-emission tomography scan demonstrates this increased glucose usage by cancer cells. This hypothesis is however disputed by the fact that cancer cells may proliferate by a mechanism outside of glucose and insulin dependence.

PATHOLOGICAL LINK BETWEEN CANCER AND DIABETES (FIG. 1)

Are There Shared Risk Factors?

The clinical scenario of patients with diabetes and cancer points to some shared risk factors. Physical inactivity and obesity are common denominators in case of cancer of the breast and endometrium. However, the link between body weight and cancer is not so clear cut (Fig. 1). Neither the Nurses Health Study nor the Bariatric Surgery Data clearly demonstrate the beneficial effect of weight loss on cancer incidence.

CANCER OF THE BREAST

Cancer of the breast is the most common malignancy in women all over the world. There is a strong link between diabetes and cancer breast. The association maybe through IGF-1 signaling pathway. Type 2 diabetes mellitus has been linked with the occurrence and progression of breast cancer in postmenopausal women.

It has been suggested that long duration diabetes may have higher incidence of breast cancer. However, the Nurses Health Study did not find this association to be strong. The tight control of diabetes has been attempted to decrease the risk of breast cancer, but this has also not been found to be useful.

Hyperglycemia may increase the growth of breast cancer, as patients with increased fasting glucose may have a higher risk of breast cancer. The number of insulin receptors is also higher in breast cancer tissues. This causes higher binding of insulin which may lead to cell proliferation. However, these hypotheses do not translate into sound epidemiological data.

The further interaction in breast cancer may be between the estrogen and insulin levels. Increased insulin levels may promote its binding to sex hormone binding globulin, releasing free estrogen which may then bind to breast cancer cells. Insulin also increases the amount of sex hormones produced from the adrenals which may predispose to the development of postmenopausal breast cancer.

Prognosis of Breast Cancer in Diabetic Women

Yanick et al. found higher mortality from breast cancer in diabetic women compared to nondiabetics. This has been further emphasized by Lipsombe et al. who showed that the mortality increases by a hazard ratio of 1.39 compared to nondiabetics. Hence, whatever be the mechanism of the association, the bad prognosis due to the confluence of these two diseases is definite.

ENDOMETRIAL CANCER

A meta-analysis of several studies showed that the relative risk for endometrial cancer in diabetics was 2.10. The common hypothesis of hyperinsulinemia and obesity along with low adiponectin levels has been found in endometrial cancer. Furthermore, recurrence of endometrial cancer is higher in diabetics and the overall prognosis is much worse.

OVARIAN CANCER

Lee et al. demonstrated a higher incidence of ovarian cancer in diabetic patients. The prognosis in patients with ovarian cancer and diabetes is also worse as studied by Bakhru et al.

Based on the hyperinsulinemia hypothesis, metformin has been tried as a preventive measure for ovarian cancer. In a study published by the Mayo clinic data from diabetic patients analyzed over 15 years, surprisingly revealed that metformin does decrease the risk of ovarian malignancies. However, this conclusion has not been substantiated by further studies and evidence falls on either side.

COLON CANCER

The Nurses Health Study with an 18-year follow-up of diabetic patients showed that there was an increased risk of colorectal cancer in diabetic women. This risk remained even after confounders such as age, body mass index, and physical inactivity were adjusted.

PANCREATIC CANCER

This cancer has probably the strongest link with diabetes with a two- to threefold higher risk compared to general population. Since pancreatic cancer can also cause diabetes establishing causality becomes more difficult.

Several theories exist for this higher incidence. The exposure of pancreatic exocrine cells to high levels of insulin has been proposed. This, however, does not explain the higher incidence in T1DM where the insulin levels are low.

LIVER CANCER

The higher incidence of hepatocellular carcinoma in diabetes mellitus may be explained through several ways. The liver is the first target of hyperinsulinemia that is evident in the portal circulation in T2DM. Further, T2DM is known to cause a higher incidence of nonalcoholic fatty liver disease. This is well known to result in cirrhosis and further predispose to hepatocellular carcinoma. However, there is no difference in the incidence between men and women.

DRUG THERAPY OF DIABETES AND CANCER

Evidence has emerged about the link between drugs used for the treatment of diabetes and cancer. It has been mooted that this could contribute to the increased incidence of cancer in diabetic patients.

Thiazolidinediones

The Cleveland Clinic Diabetes Registry computed and cross-indexed the tumor registry between 1998 and 2006 to look at the link between these two noncommunicable diseases. This study looked at the incidence of cancer in women treated with thiazolidinediones. The conclusion was a decreased incidence of cancer in women put on these drugs. However, the last word of this association is not yet concluded.

Insulins

Glargine, the basal insulin, came under a cloud because it was suspected to produce increased breast cancer in women in a study from Scotland; however, this was vetoed by another study from Sweden. The Outcome Reduction with Initial Glargine Intervention (ORIGIN) trial which used glargine found no increased incidence of breast cancer in the glargine arm putting to rest this proposed association.

CONCLUSION

In conclusion, cancer specific to women such as malignancies of ovaries, breast, and endometrium are definitely more common in diabetic women.

Physicians treating women with diabetes should routinely screen for these cancers to enable early detection and intervention. The pathological links between diabetes and cancer still need further exploration.

Research focused on such cellular mechanisms may help in the prevention of cancers in diabetic women. Furthermore, the prognosis of these cancers may also be altered by control of diabetes and may hence impact morbidity and mortality significantly.

Lastly, the effect of drugs used in diabetes and their propensity for altering the incidence of cancer are exciting areas for further research.

SUGGESTED READINGS

1. Bakhru A, Buckanovich RJ, Griggs JJ. The impact of diabetes on survival in women with ovarian cancer. Gynecol Oncol. 2011;121(1):106-11.
2. Burstein HJ, Demetri GD, Mueller E, et al. Use of the peroxisome proliferator-activated receptor (PPAR) gamma ligand troglitazone as treatment for refractory breast cancer: a phase II study. Breast Cancer Res Treat. 2003;79:391-7.
3. Colhoun HM, SDRN Epidemiology Group. Use of insulin glargine and cancer incidence in Scotland: a study from the Scottish Diabetes Research Network Epidemiology Group Diabetologia. 2009;52(9):1755-65.
4. Dikshit RP, Ramadas K, Hashibe M, et al. Association between diabetes mellitus and pre-malignant oral diseases: a cross sectional study in Kerala, India. Int J Cancer. 2006;118(2):453-7.
5. Dilokthornsakul P, Chaiyakunapruk N, Termrungruanglert W, et al. The effects of metformin on ovarian cancer: a systematic review. Int J Gynecol Cancer. 2013;23(9):1544-51.
6. Eliassen AH, Colditz GA, Rosner B, et al. Adult weight change and risk of postmenopausal breast cancer. JAMA. 2006;296:193-201.
7. Ferlay J, Soerjomataram I, Ervik M, et al. GLOBOCAN 2012 v1.0, Cancer Incidence and Mortality Worldwide: IARC CancerBase No. 11. Lyon, France: International Agency for Research on Cancer; 2013.
8. Friberg E, Orsini N, Mantzoros CS, et al. Diabetes mellitus and risk of endometrial cancer: a meta-analysis Diabetologia. 2007;50:1365-74.
9. Friedenreich CM, Orenstein MR. Physical activity and cancer prevention: etiologic evidence and biological mechanisms. J Nutr. 2002;132:3456S-3464S.
10. Giovannucci E, Harlan DM, Archer MC, et al. Diabetes and cancer: a consensus report. CA Cancer J Clin. 2010;60:207-21.
11. Johnson JA, Bowker SL. Intensive glycaemic control and cancer risk in type 2 diabetes: a meta-analysis of major trials. Diabetologia. 2011;54:25-31.
12. Lee JY, Jeon I, Kim JW, et al. Diabetes mellitus and ovarian cancer risk: a systematic review and meta-analysis of observational studies. Int J Gynecol Cancer. 2013;23(3):402-12.
13. Lipscombe LL, Goodwin PJ, Zinman B, et al. The impact of diabetes on survival following breast cancer. Breast Cancer Res Treat. 2008;109:389-95.
14. ORIGIN Trial Investigators, Gerstein HC, Bosch J, et al. Basal insulin and cardiovascular and other outcomes in dysglycemia. N Engl J Med. 2012;367:319-28.
15. Rapp K, Schroeder J, Klenk J, et al. Fasting blood glucose and cancer risk in a cohort of more than 140,000 adults in Austria. Diabetologia. 2006;49:945-52.
16. Renehan AG. Bariatric surgery, weight reduction, and cancer prevention. Lancet Oncol. 2009;10:640-1.

17. Sinha A, Kumar R, Pawar B, et al. Population-based estimation of mortality and occurrence of cancer in patients with and without diabetes in Pune. Curr Sci. 2013;105:486-91.
18. Slattery ML, Benson J, Berry TD, et al. Dietary sugar and colon cancer. Cancer Epidemiol Biomarkers Prev. 1997;6:677-85.
19. Stevens RJ, Roddam AW, Beral V. Pancreatic cancer in type 1 and young-onset diabetes: systematic review and meta-analysis. Br J Cancer. 2007;96:507-9.
20. Yancik R, Wesley MN, Ries LA, et al. Effect of age and comorbidity in postmenopausal breast cancer patients aged 55 years and older. JAMA. 2001;285:885-92.
21. Yeshaya A, Orvieto R, Dicker D, et al. Menstrual characteristics of women suffering from insulin-dependent diabetes mellitus. Int J Fertil Menopausal Stud. 1995;40:269-73.
22. Yun J, Rago C, Cheong I, et al. Glucose deprivation contributes to the development of KRAS pathway mutations in Tumor cells. Science. 2009;325:1555-9.
23. Zanders MM, Boll D, van Steenbergen LN, et al. Effect of diabetes on endometrial cancer recurrence and survival. Maturitas. 2013;74(1):37-43.
24. Zendehdel K, Nyré O, Östenson CG, et al. Cancer Incidence in Patients With Type 1 Diabetes Mellitus: A Population-Based Cohort Study in Sweden. J Natl Cancer Inst. 2003;95(23):1797-800.

24
CHAPTER

Sexual Health

Rakesh K Sahay, P Venu Madhavi

INTRODUCTION

Diabetes is one of the largest global health emergencies of 21st century. Approximately 415 million adults are estimated to have diabetes in the world out of which about 199.5 million will be women as per data published in International Diabetes Federation in 2015. By 2040, 642 million adults all over the world are estimated to suffer from diabetes. About 69.2 million people in India are suffering from diabetes, with India being second most common nation with highest prevalence. About half of adults with diabetes in India are women.

The World Psychiatric Association defines sexual health as "not merely an absence of sexual disorders, but a dynamic and harmonious state involving erotic and reproductive experiences and fulfillment, within a broader physical, emotional, interpersonal, social, and spiritual sense of well being, in a culturally informed, freely and responsibly chosen, and ethical framework."

The prevalence of female sexual dysfunction is as high as 35–60% in general population in India. About 20–80% of this occurs in women with type 2 diabetes mellitus (T2DM). Sexual dysfunction in men with diabetes is well recognized but data in women with diabetes are very scant. The main motive of this chapter is to outline various aspects of sexual health in women with diabetes which are to be detected and treated for their well being.

SEXUAL HEALTH IN WOMEN

Sexual health is an important aspect of human well being. It involves complex interactions between nervous system, endocrine system, and vascular system. It is influenced by the cultural, ethical, social, and religious factors.

Sexual health is one of the most neglected aspects in India, especially in women due to cultural and social taboos. There are also very few studies assessing sexual health in women with validated questionnaires.

THE SEXUAL RESPONSE CYCLE

Masters and Kaplan have categorized sexual response cycle as a four phase process (Figs 1 and 2):

1. Desire
2. Excitement
3. Orgasm
4. Resolution.

The first phase is characterized by motivational aspects of sexual response in which sexual urge and fantasies are included. The second phase is sexual excitement. It refers to subjective feeling of sexual pleasure and associated physiological changes. This phase in women includes vaginal lubrication. Plateauing is heightened state of excitement attained with continued stimulation. The third phase orgasm refers to peak of sexual pleasure associated with rhythmic contraction of genital musculature. This is followed by resolution.

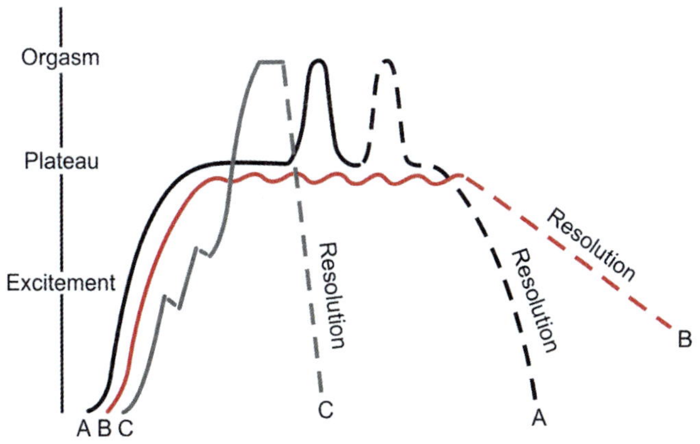

FIG. 1: Sexual response cycle in women

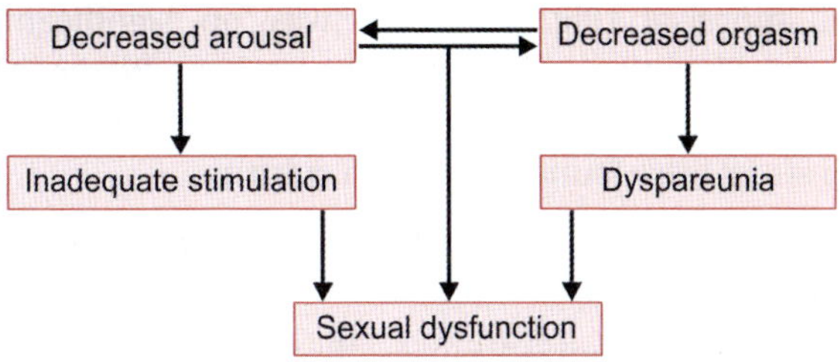

FIG. 2: Various domains of sexual response cycle affected by diabetes

SEXUAL DYSFUNCTION IN WOMEN WITH DIABETES

Type 2 diabetes mellitus is one of the most common causes affecting sexual health of a woman. Sexual dysfunction is as common as twice the rate compared to normal healthy counterparts. As T2DM occurs in the productive period of adulthood, sexual dysfunction could disrupt the stability of couple. Diabetes affects all the domains of sexual functioning.

Sexual Desire Disorder

Most of the diabetic women suffer from this disorder. Sexual urge is either diminished or reduced. Sexual fantasies and thoughts are absent.

Arousal Disorder

Up to 76% of diabetic women are affected with arousal disorder (Basson et al., 2001). They may present with reduced sexual stimulation and sensations which may be characterized by reduced vulvar swelling or vaginal lubrication. Some women may only have subjective arousal disorder where vaginal lubrication is normal but there is no sense of pleasure and excitement.

Orgasmic Disorder

Though there is arousal, this disorder is characterized by lack of orgasm or diminished intensity of orgasmic sensations or marked delay of orgasm.

Dyspareunia

Dyspareunia is characterized by recurrent or persistent pain with attempted or complete vaginal entry.

ETIOPATHOGENESIS

Factors associated with diabetes that correlates with sexual dysfunction include duration of diabetes, long-term complications, and illness-specific psychological appraisal (Fig. 3). There was no significant association between sexual dysfunction and glycemic control or adherence to treatment. Long-term complications like neuropathy and vascular causes along with psychological stress were found to be main culprits.

Psychological Issues

One of the most well-recognized causes of sexual dysfunction in women is depression. Women with T2DM are at increased risk of depression. As most

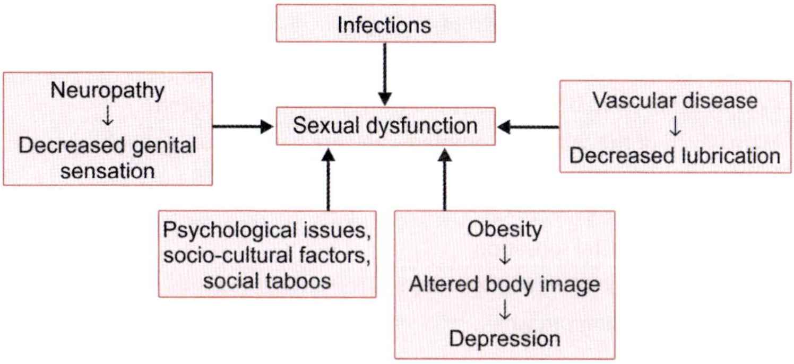

FIG. 3 Etiopathogenesis of sexual dysfunction in women with diabetes

of the women with T2DM are obese, altered body image may perpetuate sexual dysfunction, and depression. Hence, obesity, T2DM and depression make a vicious cycle.

Women who have adapted successfully to diabetes have good sexual health. Indian women with diabetes have more psychological stress and perceive higher burden of personal and social distress associated with the disease. Gender discrimination with social and cultural disparities is major culprit resulting in poor psychological well being. Lack of knowledge about disease is also one of the major contributing factors.

Peripheral Neuropathy and Vascular Causes

Peripheral neuropathy in women with T2DM can cause decreased genital sensation and arousal disorder. In some studies they have demonstrated reduced vibration sense in external genitalia in women with T2DM though it had no correlation with sexual dysfunction. Vascular compromise may result in decreased lubrication and dyspareunia.

Evaluation

Eliciting a proper history is important. Clinicians often feel uncomfortable in asking history related to sexual health. This could be because of lack of training or due to lack of time, or due to associated stigma, or embarrassment of patient or doctor. In India, cultural and social issues too play a major role.

It is always better to attend to patient discomfort by deferring sensitive questions to subsequent visit and to use an alternate terminology to provide explicit sexual details. There may be lack of time in practically assessing sexual function in clinical encounter. Thus, some clinicians use validated research instruments, i.e., there are some validated questionnaires designed to understand the degree of sexual dysfunction.

BOX 1 Sexual symptom checklist

- Are you satisfied with your sexual function? If no, please continue:
  - How long have you been dissatisfied with your sexual function?
  - Mark which of the following problems you are having and highlight the one that is most bothersome:
    - Little or no interest in sex
    - Decreased genital sensation
    - Decreased vaginal lubrication (dryness)
    - Problem reaching orgasm
    - Pain during sex
    - Other
  - Would you like to talk about this with your health care professional?

The American College of Obstetricians and Gynecologists guidelines offer a brief checklist of sexual symptoms in women (Box 1).

TOOLS TO ASSESS SEXUAL FUNCTION

Female Sexual Functioning Index

It consists of 19 questions involving six domains.

1. Questions regarding desire (two questions)
2. Arousal (four questions)
3. Lubrication (four questions)
4. Orgasm
5 Satisfaction
6. Pain (three questions each) are included in the questionnaire.

It evaluates sexual function in last 4 weeks. It is scored using Likert scale of 0–5. Women with lower scores have higher probability of sexual dysfunction.

Arizona Sexual Experience Scale

It is a 5-item scale, used as screening tool for female sexual dysfunction. It includes five domains:

1. Sex drive
2. Arousal
3. Vaginal lubrication
4. Orgasm
5. Satisfaction following orgasm.

Each item is scored from 1 to 6 with each score having a brief, simple anchor. It evaluates sexual functioning in the past week including on the day of interview.

The total score is from 5–30. Sexual dysfunction is defined as:

- Total 19 or more, or
- 5 or more on any item, or
- 4 or more on 3 items.

TOOLS TO ASSESS PSYCHOLOGICAL ISSUES

The Appraisal of Diabetes Scale

It is a 7-item self-report scale used for assessing the individual's appraisal of his or her diabetes in terms of his or her thoughts about diabetes. Respondents rate each statement on a 5 point Likert scale. The Appraisal of Diabetes Scale (ADS) can be incisive as a quick 5 minute screening tool to examine a patient's adjustment to diabetes. The test is simple to score and interpret. Strong correlation between ADS and anxiety, and anger and diabetes-associated hassles has been found. The scale reflects four components:

1. Emotional disturbance
2. Coping
3. Loss of control
4. Consequences of diabetes which is assessed by seven questions scored 1–5 in Likert scale with maximum score being 33 and minimum being 7. Lesser score indicates positive attitude toward disease.

Hospital Anxiety and Depression Scale

Hospital Anxiety and Depression Scale is a brief widely used screening tool to measure psychological stress. It consists of 14 items and consists of two subscales: anxiety and depression. Each item is rated based on a 4-point scale. Maximum score is 21 for both subscales. Scores 0–7 on either subscale are considered normal and those equal to or above 11 are considered to have significant psychological morbidity. Scores between 8 and 10 indicate a borderline status.

TREATMENT

Recognition and multidisciplinary management of sexual dysfunction would be of great benefits for women with diabetes. It has to be treated by both pharmacologic and nonpharmacologic means (Box 2).

Nonpharmacologic Therapy (Box 3)

A proper counseling is very important part of therapy as most of the Indian diabetic women suffer from anxiety and depression. The five Es of sexual counseling are:

1. Experience

BOX 2 Treatment of individual domains

Disorder of sexual desire
- Antidepressants
- Psychosexual therapy
- Couple centered care
- Testosterone

Arousal disorder
- Genital vibrators
- Clitoral devices
- Lubricants like water-based gels
- Phosphodiesterase 5 inhibitors
- Oral contraceptive pills

Disorders of orgasm
- Genital vibrators
- Clitoral devices
- Pelvic exercises
- Psychosexual therapy

Dyspareunia
- Vaginal dilatation
- Arousal enhancement
- Kegel's exercises

BOX 3 Nonpharmacologic therapy
- Physical exercise
- Relaxation therapy
- Yoga
- Cognitive behavioral therapy
- Healthy diet
- Pelvic exercises

2. Etiquette
3. Empathy
4. Ethnic
5. Cultural understanding and environment conducive for relaxation.

A healthy diet forms an important part of counseling for female sexual dysfunction. These women must be advised to take diet rich in vitamins and minerals and if required nutraceuticals should to be advised. Smoking and alcoholism to be avoided.

Physical Activity

Moderate physical activity is advised at least thrice a week. Sexual fitness will be achieved only when one is physically fit. Yoga can be advised in which certain "Asanas" increase pelvic blood flow and, thereby, improve sexual function.

Cognitive Behavioral Therapy

Cognitive behavioral therapy plays an important role in improving sexual dysfunction. A multimodal cognitive behavioral approach entails sexual intimacy exercises, sensate focus, communication skills training, emotional skills training, reinforcement training, and cognitive restructuring.

Other modes of therapy like relaxation therapy, vivid imagery, Master and Johnson's therapy, gradual desensitization, and pelvic floor exercises can be tried.

Couple centered care can be given. Counseling of both partners is sometimes required to achieve desired outcome.

PHARMACOLOGIC THERAPY

Disorder of Desire

Depressive illness should be treated with antidepressants. Psychosexual support is to be given. Couple therapy has been proven to improve partner intimacy. Testosterone is the principal treatment for sexual desire disorder.

Disorder of Arousal

Use of vibrators has been found to be useful in improving arousal disorder. Encouraging adequate foreplay to increase stimulation may be useful. Localized aids can be used which create gentle vacuum for the clitoris and increase genital blood flow and sensitivity.

Pharmacological treatment is found to be useful but it cannot be used on a regular basis and they are not curative. Nitric oxide enhancers, i.e., phosphodiesterase type 5 inhibitors such as sildenafil and tadalafil can be used. Nitric oxide mediated smooth muscle relaxation causes vasodilation and improves lubrication and vulval engorgement. Estrogen-containing vaginal creams, phentolamine, prostaglandin E, and L-arginine are also useful in arousal disorder.

Orgasmic Disorder

Treatment mainly includes positive sexual attitudes and fantasy training. Vibrating sex aids and clitoral devices can be used. Kegel's exercises can be done to facilitate easier orgasms. Sensate exercises to reduce anxiety are also found to be useful.

Dyspareunia

Vaginal dilatation is the oldest method used to treat dyspareunia. Kegel's exercises with certain relaxation exercises can be practiced. Arousal enhancement improves dyspareunia.

CONCLUSION

Sexual dysfunction is an age old complication associated with diabetes in men. Female sexual dysfunction is also as common as it is in men with T2DM. Though we are in 21st century, still social taboos and restrictions have resulted in negligence of sexual health in women. Physicians must give attention to sexual health when evaluating any case of T2DM. A secure environment should be provided in the clinic so that patient feels comfortable to disclose the issues. Doctors should be trained appropriately in this field to improve patient care for the social and psychological well-being.

SUGGESTED READINGS

1. Abu Ali RM, Al Hajeri RM, Khader YS, et al. Sexual dysfunction in Jordanian diabetic women. Diabetes Care. 2008;31:1580-1.
2. Anil Kumar MN, Pai NB, Nanjegowda RB, et al. Etiology and management of sexual dysfunction. Online J Health Allied Sci. 2009;8:1.
3. Bajaj S, Jawad F, Islam N, et al. South Asian women with diabetes: psychosocial challenges and management: consensus statement. Indian J Endocrinol Metab. 2013;17:548-62.
4. Bargiota A, Dimitropoulos K, Tzortzis V, et al. Sexual dysfunction in diabetic women. Hormones. 2011;10:196-206.
5. Dogra A, Tharoor H, Muttineni K. Sexual dysfunction in females. In: Kar N, Kar GC (Eds). Comprehension Textbook of Sexual Medicine. New Delhi: Jaypee Brothers; 2005. pp. 154-65.
6. International Diabetes Federation. IDF Diabetes Atlas, 7th edition. Brussels, Belgium: International Diabetes Federation; 2015.
7. Kalra B, Kalra S, Chawla K, et al. Sexual attitudes, knowledge and function of women with diabetes. Internet J Geriatr Gerontol. 2010;5(2).
8. Katon W, Maj M, Sartorius N. Depression and Diabetes. Italy: Wiley; 2010.
9. Magnuson S, Collins S. Collaboration between couples, counselors and physical therapists when treating dyspareunia: an untapped partnership. Fam J. 2002;10:109-111.
10. Mezzich JE, Hernandez-Serrano R (Eds). Comprehensive treatment of specific sexual disorders. Psychiatry and Sexual Health: An Integrative Approach. Lanham: Jason Aronson, Inc.; 2006. pp. 149-70.
11. Mezzich JE, Hernandez-Serrano R (Eds). World Health Organization's statement on sexual health (2002). Psychiatry and Sexual Health: An Integrative Approach. Lanham: Jason Aronson, Inc.; 2006. pp. 186-8.
12. Mills L. Sexual and reproductive health in women with diabetes. J Diabetes Nurs. 2015;19:272-5.
13. Nagpal M, Jangid R. A study of sexual function in women with type 2 diabetes mellitus in a tertiary care centre in India. J Psychiatry. 2016;19(6):393.
14. Ogbera A, Chinenye S, Akinlade A, et al. FMCP Frequency and correlates of sexual dysfunction in women with diabetes mellitus. J Sex Med. 2009;6:3401-6.
15. O'Donnell O. Access to health care in developing countries: breaking down demand side barriers. Cad Saude Publica. 2007;23:2820-34.
16. Park K, Ahn K, Chang JS, et al. Diabetes induced alteration of clitoral hemodynamics and structure in the rabbit. J Urol. 2002;168:1269-72.
17. Reis SL, Abdo CH. Benefits and risks of testosterone treatment for hypoactive sexual desire disorder in women: a critical review of studies published in the decades preceding and succeeding the advent of phosphodiesterase type 5 inhibitors. Clinics (Sao Paulo). 2014;69:294-303.
18. Rockliffe-Fidler C, Kiemle G. Sexual function in diabetic women: a psychological perspective. Sex Relat Ther. 2003;18:143.
19. Sathyanarana Rao TS, Nagaraj AM. Female sexuality. Indian J Psychiatry. 2015;57:296-302.
20. Trudel G, Marchand A, Ravart M, et al. The effect of cognitive behavioural group treatment program on hypoactive sexual desire women. Sex Relat Ther. 2001;16:146-64.
21. Vafaeimanesh J, Raei M, Hosseinzadeh F, et al. Evaluation of sexual dysfunction in women with type 2 diabetes. Indian J Endocrinol Metab. 2014;18(2):175-9.

25
CHAPTER

Anxiety and Depression

Yatan PS Balhara, Arghya Pal, Sanjay Kalra

INTRODUCTION

Diabetes mellitus is one of the leading causes of mortality and morbidity worldwide. The prevalence of diabetes mellitus worldwide is 8.3%. The Indian studies estimate the prevalence to be around 9.3%. In 2013, about 65 million people between 20 and 79 years in India were found to be suffering from diabetes mellitus. By 2035, this number has been predicted to reach 109 million.

Individuals with diabetes mellitus have been shown to be at a higher risk of developing mental health comorbidities as compared to general population, amongst which depression, anxiety disorder, and eating disorder have been found to be the most common. These comorbidities have been found to have a profound effect on the course of the illness. This includes issue of complications secondary to diabetes mellitus and therapeutic adherence. The current chapter is focused at addressing the comorbidity of depressive and anxiety disorders among women diagnosed with diabetes mellitus. Evidence shows that there is no difference in the prevalence of diabetes mellitus across the genders. However, there are certain issues relevant to this theme that are unique to women. The current chapter is aimed at addressing the women specific issues pertinent to depression and anxiety disorders co-occurring with diabetes mellitus.

EPIDEMIOLOGY

Studies on the prevalence of the psychiatric disorders exclusively among women with diabetes mellitus have been relatively scarce. Studies have shown that the chances of developing mental disorders among women lifespan after developing diabetes mellitus is about twice as that of normal population. In a study done on clinical population with type 2 diabetes mellitus (T2DM), around 32% and 22% patients met the cutoff for anxiety and depressive disorders, respectively when evaluated by Hospital Anxiety and Depression Scale (HADS). However, the figures increase further up to 60% and 53% when the symptoms of anxiety and depression are evaluated using HADS in patients with type 1 diabetes mellitus (T1DM). Another study that included data from a cohort of 90,686 patients (59% females) showed that depression was more prevalent among patients with diagnosed and undiagnosed diabetes mellitus as opposed to patients without diabetes mellitus, whereas anxiety was prevalent more in patients who were aware that they have been diagnosed with diabetes mellitus. In a study done on females with newly diagnosed, untreated endocrine disorders, it was found that the prevalence of major depressive disorder and anxiety disorders using Structured Clinical Interview for Axis I-Patient Edition (SCID-P) in diabetes mellitus were around 12% and 10%, respectively. In another study exclusively on female patients with diabetes mellitus, it was found that about 33% and 50% of the respondents reported of depressive and anxiety disorder, respectively using the Composite International Diagnostic Interview. A meta-analysis showed that the odds of developing comorbid depression was significantly higher amongst women in uncontrolled studies (versus controlled studies) and in a clinical settings (as opposed to a community sample). In a systematic review conducted on the prevalence of anxiety disorders in patients with diabetes, generalized anxiety disorder was found in 14% of the patients and 40% of the patients reported elevated symptoms of anxiety. The symptoms of anxiety were also found to be significantly higher among females as compared to males (55.3% vs. 32.9%, $p < 0.0001$).

PATHOPHYSIOLOGICAL MECHANISMS

The relationship between diabetes, anxiety, and depression has been one of the most intriguing topics of research. The search for a common genetic factor contributing to the illnesses has been dismal for both T1DM and T2DM. However, there has been encouraging results in the search for the epigenetic basis for the same. A key candidate for the common explanation has been dysfunction in the stress system. It has been postulated that chronic stress leads to activation of the hypothalamo-pituitary-adrenal axis (HPA axis) and the sympathetic nervous system (SNS). Chronic hypercortisolemia which occurs in response to chronic stress, and chronic SNS stimulation leads to insulin resistance which finally results in T2DM. Chronic stress, on the other hand, also causes dysfunction of the limbic system and disturbs neurogenesis of the hippocampal region, which is implicated in depression.

Moreover, chronic stress also causes immunological dysfunction causing release of the proinflammatory cytokines. This, on one hand, causes dysfunction of the pancreatic β-cells, leading to diabetes mellitus, and also causes depression due to disruption of the neurotransmitter metabolism, neuroendocrine function, and synaptic plasticity. This explanation has been especially implicated in the pathogenesis of the T1DM.

RELATIONSHIP BETWEEN DIABETES MELLITUS AND DEPRESSION

- Diabetic risk in patients with depressive disorders: It has been established that the risk of developing diabetes mellitus is higher in patients with depression. Similar findings have also been replicated in studies that have been conducted only among women. In women, depression increases the chances of insulin resistance mainly causing central obesity. Patients with diabetes have a higher risk of having a complicated course of depression characterized by suicidality and hospitalizations. Other than the mechanisms referred above, another aspect that has been implicated is use of multiple antidepressant subclasses that has been associated with suboptimal glycemic control (Table 1)
- Depression risk in patients with diabetes: It has been stated that patients with undiagnosed diabetes mellitus has a higher prevalence of depression. Various lifestyle factors like sedentary lifestyle, unhealthy diet has been deemed as contributory. The available evidence also points out that the risk of suicidality is also higher in patients with diabetes mellitus and is associated with a higher fatality, though there is some evidence to the contrary. Other than that, a strong association has also been found between the depression and use of oral hypoglycemic

Table 1: Grouping of various psychotropic medications based on fetal safety and impact on glycemia control

Adverse effect on developing fetus based on FDA category	Impact on glycemia control	
	Little impact	High impact
FDA category C	• Fluoxetine • Sertraline • Citalopram • Escitalopram • Venlafaxine • Duloxetine • Bupropion	• Venlafaxine • Fluvoxamine • Mirtazapine • Tetracyclic antidepressants (amitriptyline, nortriptyline)
FDA category D	–	• MAOI (phenelzine, tranylcypromine, and isocarboxazid) • Paroxetine

FDA, Food and Drug Administration; MAOI, monoamine oxidase inhibitor.

drugs. But use of insulin, on the other hand, has been shown to improve the symptoms of depression. Diabetes also causes microvascular damage to the organs leading to reduction of size in various parts of the brain. Studies have been able to show that there is an inverse relationship between the glycemic control and volume of hippocampus, the latter of which is also seen in depression

- A longitudinal 10-year follow-up study conducted on 65,381 females aged between 50 and 75 years, tried to establish the direction of association of the relationship between diabetes mellitus and depression. The study found that as the severity of the depressive symptoms increased, the risk of developing diabetes mellitus increased. Likewise, the risk of developing depression also increased as the presentation of diabetes mellitus in the patients became severer, controlling for all the covariates.

The presence of depression plays a synergistic role in the course of diabetes by increasing the risk of both microvascular and macrovascular complications. Presence of depression also leads to early onset of the complications and leads to worsening of the quality of life. However, depression continues to be underdiagnosed and untreated. This co-occurrence among women living with diabetes also leads to increased healthcare use and higher expenditures.

RELATIONSHIP BETWEEN DIABETES MELLITUS AND ANXIETY DISORDERS

- Risk of anxiety in patients with diabetes: A number of studies have identified the higher risk of developing anxiety disorders in patients with diabetes. A large scale telephone-based survey conducted on 217,379 respondents showed that the patients with a self-disclosed diagnosis of diabetes reported a higher prevalence of lifetime diagnosis of anxiety disorders. Another multi-country study found that the prevalence of anxiety disorders were significantly more in patients of diabetes as compared to the nondiabetic population. However, a study conducted among newly diagnosed cases of T1DM failed to replicate this trend and found that the risk was no greater than the reference population
- There are commonly two points in the course of diabetes when the symptoms of anxiety increase; first, when the patient becomes aware of the diagnosis and, second, when the complications of diabetes sets in. Anxiety disorders also complicate the course of diabetes in various ways. The symptoms of anxiety disorders overlap with that of hypoglycemia which often leads to delay in diagnosis of both conditions and mismanagement. Patients with specific phobias about needle

prick or blood may have a surge in anxiety symptoms when they are diagnosed or are prescribed parenteral therapy. Finally, in many cases fear of hypoglycemia may lead to patients maintaining a higher blood glucose level and becoming noncompliant to the set treatment goals.

SPECIAL ISSUES IN FEMALES

A chronic illness like diabetes is bound to share a complex relationship with the various psychosocial issues associated with the female gender. A study conducted among women living with diabetes in India showed that presence of depressive symptoms translated to poorer control of their glycemic status. However, in spite of that the women lacked the psychological distress and continued to fulfill their social roles. The explanatory model suggested by the authors speculated that the women in this group maintained participation in their culturally valued roles which may play a buffering role for their mental health. Such findings, to some extent, have also been replicated in the African-American population using a qualitative approach. It has been postulated that African-American mothers with diabetes mellitus are exposed to a number of stressors and are required to employ exaggerated coping strategies to prove their worth leading to "Superwoman Syndrome". Such coping strategies often may be adaptive, enabling the mothers to adopt a positive outlook toward the challenge. However, often it may be maladaptive (avoidant, denial, anger, etc.) which leads to a poor individual adjustment and poor clinical outcome.

Another important issue that requires discussion is the journey of the women living with diabetes mellitus through pregnancy. Various psychosocial issues crop up at this stage like increased levels of anxiety, distress, and also a sense of discontentment owing to the overtly clinical approach focused on management of the complications of diabetes as opposed to a positive journey toward motherhood. It is suggested that these issues to be countered by establishing a trusting relationship with the healthcare professionals, sharing experiences, and involving the patients in decision making. However, very little attention is paid to these details in clinical practice.

Both anxiety and depressive symptoms are more commonly prevalent among patients with diabetes mellitus approaching menopause. A study conducted among Malaysian population with T2DM showed that the level of anxiety and depressive symptoms were higher in menopausal women with diabetes as compared to population without diabetes, which adversely affected the quality of life of the patients. Though the presentation of menopause remained same across both diagnosed with diabetes and controls, the chances of developing psychological symptoms increased when the severity of physical or vasomotor symptoms increased.

MANAGEMENT

Most authors suggest a balanced approach to the management of diabetes mellitus co-occurring with depression and anxiety, where emphasis should be placed equally on the glycemic control and the alleviation of the psychological problems. The treatment of psychiatric comorbidity does not necessarily translate in to better glycemic control. It has been found that other factors like duration of the illness, presence of complications, and initial management of diabetes play an important role in the final outcome of the treatment.

There has been substantial evidence that advocates that patients with diabetes mellitus should be screened for the presence of any psychological symptoms, particularly depression and anxiety. The most widely used instrument in this regard is the HADS. However, other scales that have been used in this regard include Beck Depression Inventory and Centre for Epidemiologic Studies Depression scale.

When any psychiatric comorbidity is detected in diabetes mellitus, the focus should be to treat both the disorders at the same time. The mainstay of treatment for depressive and anxiety symptoms in diabetes mellitus continues to be antidepressants and psychological interventions. The most commonly used antidepressants include the serotonin reuptake inhibitors (SSRIs) and the tricyclic antidepressants (TCAs). There has been a furor over the deleterious effects of the antidepressants. Studies have suggested that, on a short-term, antidepressant therapy leads to an improvement in the insulin sensitivity. However, on a long-term, the antidepressants, particularly TCAs, may lead to impaired insulin sensitivity. Pregnancy poses an added challenge in the choice of pharmacological agents for the management of psychiatric issues cropping up (Table 1).

There has been a considerable research on the effectiveness of the various nonpharmacological modalities in general population. The most rewarding therapies include cognitive behavioral therapy (CBT) and self-management training. Cognitive behavioral therapy has shown to result in reduction of the blood glucose levels and also improvement in individual and family functioning. Self-management training which often included exercise-based interventions, has shown to produce improvement in the quality of life. A specialized program which was developed for depression in women with diabetes, used group therapy based on the principles of CBT and was found to be effective in treatment for both the conditions.

Hormone replacement therapy (HRT) has been associated with better glycemic control in patients with diabetes. It has also been used for management of the psychological symptoms in patients with menopause. However, there has been a reciprocal increase in the use of antidepressants for the control of the psychological symptoms after the concern of potential harm of using estrogen monotherapy as HRT.

CONCLUSION

Anxiety and depression are among the most frequent psychiatric comorbidities in patients with diabetes. This co-occurrence has a deleterious effect with regards to the willingness for treatment, decision-making, therapeutic adherence, course, and outcome. The treatment of the psychiatric comorbidities remains of utmost importance among women living with diabetes.

SUGGESTED READINGS

1. Bădescu SV, Tătaru C, Kobylinska L, et al. The association between Diabetes mellitus and Depression. J Med Life. 2016;9(2):120-5.
2. Balhara YP. Diabetes and psychiatric disorders. Indian J Endocrinol Metab. 2011;15(4):274-83.
3. Collins MM, Corcoran P, Perry IJ. Anxiety and depression symptoms in patients with diabetes. Diabet Med J Br Diabet Assoc. 2009;26(2):153-61.
4. Ducat L, Philipson LH, Anderson BJ. The mental health comorbidities of diabetes. JAMA. 2014;312(7):691-2.
5. Gale EA, Gillespie KM. Diabetes and gender. Diabetologia. 2001;44(1):3-15.
6. Pan A, Lucas M, Sun Q, et al. Bidirectional association between depression and type 2 diabetes mellitus in women. Arch Intern Med. 2010;170(21):1884-91.
7. Penckofer SM, Ferrans C, Mumby P, et al. A Psychoeducational Intervention (SWEEP) for Depressed Women with Diabetes. Ann Behav Med Publ Soc Behav Med. 2012;44(2):192-206.
8. Rubin RR, Ma Y, Marrero DG, et al. Elevated depression symptoms, antidepressant medicine use, and risk of developing diabetes during the diabetes prevention program. Diabetes Care. 2008;31(3):420-6.
9. Samuel-Hodge CD, Headen SW, Skelly AH, et al. Influences on day-to-day self-management of type 2 diabetes among African-American women: spirituality, the multi-caregiver role, and other social context factors. Diabetes Care. 2000;23(7):928-33.
10. Sarkar S, Balhara YP. Diabetes mellitus and suicide. Indian J Endocrinol Metab. 2014;18(4):468-74.

26
CHAPTER

Impact on Women: Having a Family Member with Diabetes

Sanjay Agarwal, Shruti V Sheth

INTRODUCTION

Chronic illnesses have a way of creeping into the lives of not only the victims but also the family members. The uncertainty associated with chronic illnesses exposes the family to great levels of stress. Continuous fear of adverse symptoms, complications, and consequent hospital admissions plague the minds of not only the patients but also the family. Even in the absence of any obvious symptoms or signs, there is a never ending issue of medical, dietary, and lifestyle compliance that the patient has to follow. The care taker of the individual is thus burdened with not only the patient medications and regular follow ups but also with the patient behavior and compliance. Studies have now and again shown that the caregivers of the patient are emotionally affected not by the patient but by the illness per se. These caregivers often play a major role in a successful patient care and thus proper strategies are required to identify their needs and solve their issues.

The prevalence of diabetes is increasing rapidly and diabetes is no longer a disease of the elderly. In fact the Asian population has shown an early development of diabetes and the metabolic syndrome. Major contributors to this association are the dietary changes along with sedentary lifestyle leading to the characteristic Asian phenotype. The presence of disease in a younger population pose a major threat for the development of diabetes related complications because they have a longer duration of life with diabetes to be spent. These patients also form the major part of the driving economy of the household and the country consequently. They tend to have poor compliance, poor metabolic control, less regular follow-up rates, etc. Management of such individuals becomes an important task for the caretaker. Diabetes and the metabolic syndrome specifically is a lifestyle disorder, the management of which requires a major lifestyle modification in terms of a strict diet, healthy exercise routine, and regular follow ups.

EFFECT OF CHRONIC ILLNESSES ON QUALITY OF LIFE

Effect of family quality of life (QOL) is not an extensively studied subject. However, this is an area of healthcare that has a direct relation with the quality of disease management of the patient. When an individual is diagnosed with a chronic illness, the whole family actually suffers from the results of it. The regular schedule of the family has to be altered, prevention aspects have to be thought about for the family members, financial aspects have to be taken into consideration, etc. A large scale multispecialty study was conducted targeting key points of the QOL of family. They studied the effects of a chronic illness on emotional impact, daily activities, family relationships, sleep and health, holidays, involvement in healthcare and medical support given to family members, work and study, financial impact, social life, and time planning. The family members often have to hide their feelings from the patient and this gives an emotional impact of the illness on the family. The financial impact and work are other major issues that the family has to manage. Often, the patient has to take long leaves in their jobs in view of adverse complications. This hampers the income and also burdens the family with additional hospital and medication expenses. These conditions worsen when the patient suffers from not just one illness or disorder but also with associated comorbidities. Financial impact also had an effect on the family's social life as it prevented them from holidays and other social events. Economic distress reduces the family's ability as a whole to cope with the chronic illness.

ROLE OF A WOMAN IN THE INDIAN FAMILY

Women have received great importance in the Indian history. They are the pioneers of the nation. They form the glue of the family and keep it together. A woman assumes multiple roles in her entire life as a daughter, sister, wife, mother, daughter-in-law, etc. among many others. She basically manages the entire household with her leadership and fine administrative skills. Also, women have always been the ones providing informal care of sick family members due to various society and cultural views throughout the world.

Indian ladies have even come forward out of their homes and taken up important challenges at work and are at par with their male counterparts. However, their duties at home still continue to remain the same. Even today, they are required to accomplish all their household goals of being a wife, daughter, daughter-in-law, and mother in addition to their career oriented work schedules and deadlines. The elderly in the home depend on her both physically and emotionally for their daily care and needs. The children at home require their mother for their daily school works if not for other extracurricular classes and other training sessions. The husband also requires constant support and help in his responsibilities. To top it all, if any of the family members fall sick, it is the major duty of the lady to aid the ill.

With all the many responsibilities that a woman is challenged with, when there is a chronic illness in the family, it adds an additional burden for her. She has to fix and attend appointments with doctors, keep a check on regular medications, maintain healthcare at home, and take precautionary measures for the family among many others. Studies in the past have shown that multiple roles lead to increased stress and strain due to work overload and inter-role conflicts.

Stress coping theories claim that women caregivers are more likely to suffer from physical and mental strain related to caring for the sick and their way of coping with it also differs at large from the male caregivers. They tend to experience greater mental and physical strain.

DIABETES AFFECTING DIFFERENT MEMBERS OF THE FAMILY—ELDERLY, SPOUSE, CHILDREN

Diabetes in the Elderly

Management of diabetes in the elderly at home is a daunting task for the caretaker as there are a number of factors involved in safe and successful management. Older adults with diabetes may be new onset or long standing. Comorbidities and complications like cardiovascular disease and peripheral vascular disease and retinopathy tend to have a greater impact on the elderly patients. An elderly diabetic developing cardiovascular disease has higher cardiovascular mortality and morbidity. Apart from those, they are more prone to silent myocardial infarction, hypoglycemia, and strokes. Retinopathy leading to blindness or decreased vision greatly hampers their quality of life. The different aspects of care required are discussed.

Psychological and Emotional Support

Elderly people require constant emotional care and support from the family. Moreover, the fact that they are unable to function independently cause them to go into depression. They consider themselves to be a burden on the family. Therefore it becomes important for them to be kept engaged in different activities and in an environment where they are felt loved and cared for. Amongst all the members of the family the major responsibility for this effect lies with the caretaker. The caregiver may face various challenges like interpersonal disputes regarding medication and glucose monitoring compliance, severe anxiety associated with the prevention of different emergencies and their subsequent treatment and anxiety over progression of complications associated with diabetes.

Routine Medical Care

Diabetes is associated with many morbidities and complications. They are particularly prone to hypoglycemia, cardiovascular events, peripheral artery disease, retinopathy, etc. Prevention of these can be achieved by regular home care. They have to be examined regularly for their blood sugars, feet care, oral medications, insulin injections, and pain management. Regular visits to their doctor also forms a part of the routine medical care. Many a times, the patients may be unwilling to visit the doctor or follow any particular advice given to them by the doctor. The duty of the caretaker is to counsel and do the needful.

Usually the caregiver for an elderly patient is either his wife or a daughter-in-law who manages their daily routine. Both these groups of individuals have highlighted out different reasons of caregiver stress according to a study. The spouses indicated, their own physical abilities caused them stress while the daughters identified the responsibilities apart from the caregiving that gave them stress. However, the caregiving was comparable between the two groups.

Diabetes in Children

Diabetes is one of the most common chronic illnesses observed in children. In fact, along with type 1 diabetes mellitus (T1DM), type 2 diabetes mellitus (T2DM) is also being increasingly observed in the children due to detrimental lifestyle. Educating a child regarding diabetes and the different aspects of management is a difficult process. These children have a greater risk of morbidities and complications early in their age as they have a longer duration of diabetes to live with. Dietary and lifestyle modifications will help in regulating diabetes in T2DM children, however, the T1DM kids require adequate food and nutrition required for their growth and development. Puberty causes a disarray of hormones leading to further fluctuations of glycemias.

Major role of caregiving and management is played by the children's mothers. Having a child with diabetes has a huge psychological impact on the mother. She experiences all kinds of emotions of sadness, guilt, frustrations, etc. while caring for her child. A constant parent-child teamwork is to be undertaken for the successful management of diabetes in children.

Achievement of good metabolic and glycemic control has shown to have a positive impact on both the child and the mother. The psycho-social impact of good metabolic control on the family has been extensively studied. On the other hand when the metabolic control is not sufficient, children mainly complain of diabetes related symptoms of polyuria, polydipsia, polyphagia which also affects the QOL and the self-image for the individual kid. Parents have observed a negative effect of diabetes on the routine lives of these children. This especially affects the pubertal child as the hormonal changes along with the presence of uncontrolled diabetes prove to be a bad combination for them. Study related stress is one of the major factor hindering the adequate medical management of the teenage child.

In all these cases, the mother has to look after the overall physical, psychological, social, and educational aspects of the child and provide optimum care. Providing a balanced diet that adequately supplies nutrition for growth, managing medicine/insulin and monitoring related compliance, monitoring academic progress, providing an emotional support, and care platform are some of the major aspects of patient care when being a mother of a diabetic child. This in itself forms a major stress factor for the mother.

Management of T1DM requires constant vigilance. Parents are constantly faced with challenging conditions for optimum growth and development of their child along with the herculean task of managing diabetes. The constant fear of hypoglycemias and ketoacidosis and other complications form the major aspects of their life. The child at its every phase of growth and development faces new circumstances and resulting conditions that would then require to completely reanalyze the ongoing management strategies.

Studies have shown all these factors causing constant psychological stress to the parent. This adversely affects their own overall mental and physical health. Constant thoughts regarding the patient care leads to continued depression and guilt. This has a great impact on parent to child communication and psychological effect on the child. Many studies have been done to analyze the psychosocial impact of diabetes on the parents and especially the mothers. A quantitative analysis showed parental depression in the range of 10–74% at diagnosis amongst which 19% parents reported mental distress at 1–4 years after diagnosis.

Diabetes in Spouse

It is always frightening to realize the diagnosis and long-term disease related effects of diabetes of a loved one. The husband is considered as the head of the family in most families even today. When he gets diagnosed with diabetes or any diabetes-related complication, the family comes to a standstill. When the main earner of the family faced with these challenges, it becomes the duty of the wife to support and care and maintain him and the family. Even though the disease per se has been diagnosed in the husband, the whole family is affected by it. It is even more frightening when they develop diabetes related complications and continued morbidity. At this point, the disease has an immediate effect on the relationship of the couple. Negative effects such as depression, frustration, and guilt are faced by both the partners. This has also proven to have an adverse effect in the management of diabetes. In such circumstances, if the patient becomes careless of his health due to any reason like work, indifference, or anger, it can lead to further stress and strain for the partner.

Co-operation and understanding is of utmost importance between the husband and wife. Meal timing need to be fixed, physical activity goals to be achieved, blood glucose monitoring, and medication adherence form the important medical related aspects of life. Other aspects related to family life, career, and finance need to be balanced and arranged. Finance is another most important factor when the bread earner is faced with diabetes related complications like cardiovascular event, peripheral artery disease, etc. Apart from the routine home costs, hospital, medicine, and other miscellaneous costs need to be anticipated and arranged.

The presence of diabetic complications, be it acute or chronic, has a lasting impact on the woman's life. Studies have shown that an acute episode of severe hypoglycemia in the spouse cause more fear of hypoglycemia and related mortality, diabetes management related conflicts, and strain in marital relationship. An important diabetic complication that causes increased frustration and strain in the relationship is the occurrence of sexual dysfunction. Erectile dysfunction causes lots of diabetes related psychological distress for both the patient and the spouse and in turn greatly impacts their QOL.

Many studies have been done to quantify the number of spouses facing depression and regular stress due to having partners with diabetes. Depression and anxiety have shown to be equally present or even higher in the spouses as compared to the diabetic patients. Another study concluded that a type of synergy is present between the patient and spouse illness representations.

IMPACT OF DIABETES CARE ON THE WOMAN

Caregivers of diabetic patients are mostly women as has been observed among the various studies. It has been observed that the QOL of caregivers of T2DM patients was better than those of caregivers of T1DM patients. Various aspects are responsible for these differences. Type 1 diabetic patients are usually kids and their mothers tend to be under constant stress regarding their health. Some of them have to quit their jobs and leave their other responsibilities just for the better care of the child. Regular daily multiple insulin injections cause a sense of guilt in the mothers. Type 1 diabetic patients are usually diagnosed when they suffer from diabetic ketoacidosis for which they have to be hospitalized. Thus, the fear of acute complications and its management is constantly clouding their thought processes. In comparison to this, T2DM onset and subsequent management is a smooth process that requires good lifestyle modifications and medication adherence for weight loss and diabetes management. The stress faced by the caregiver here is more related to prevention of chronic complications and comorbidities.

It has been seen that educated and working married women caregivers who do not have any medical ailments themselves enjoy a better QOL. The longer the duration of patient illness, the lower is the QOL of the caregiver. Most of the time goes in the activities of daily living and supervision of the patient family member, be it an elderly patient, child, or a spouse.

Another major factor adding up to the caregiver stress is the basic cultural and ethnic background. This determines the support she will get from the rest of the family, and the patient support. The interpersonal relationships in the family form an important deciding factor for the caregiver stress. A family where the woman is a housewife who is responsible for managing the entire household, right from the daily household chores up to the management of the family along with the responsibility of the diabetic member has shown to have a more detrimental effect on the physical and mental health. Such ladies tend to avoid personal care, have a lower health status, and are more depressed. They are constantly burdened with the thoughts of patient care and management and often burden themselves with guilt in case of any kind of acute or chronic complication development. Often the rest of the family also holds her responsible for such incidences.

The patient response to diabetes is another factor that has the potential to cause caregiver strain. A noncompliant stubborn patient adds to the already existing load of the caregiver. The lady has to then suffer constant conflicts and persuasion for medication compliance, diet adherence, physical activity routine, and diabetes monitoring. Caregiver strain occurs due to increased demands of the patients. The number of diabetes management tasks that the caregiver is responsible for is directly linked to the amount of caregiver strain experienced.

Caregiver strain refers to the specific demands, responsibilities, difficulty, and negative psychic consequences of caring of relatives with special needs. Caregiver strain and mental health symptoms often predict each other. Among the different variable influencing caregiver strain are patient mental health, use of other outpatient services, and metabolic control. Among the other factors, family support and involvement forms one of the major determinants of caregiver psychological health as discussed above.

CONCLUSION

The Indian woman forms the building block of her home and the society. Her health in terms of physical, mental, and social well-being is very important for the proper functioning of the household. Women caregiver health has been given very little attention in the past. Caregiver stress and strain are very less thought of and they end up being the silent sufferers of the chronic illness in the family. An increased awareness at all levels from the doctor to the family can help in improving the standard of care of the caregivers. This will subsequently have a major impact in the patient medical management and outcomes too.

SUGGESTED READINGS

1. Anderson BJ, Miller JP, Auslander WF, et al. Family characteristics of diabetic adolescents: Relationship to metabolic control. Diabetes Care. 1981;4(6):586-94.

2. Aranda MP, Knight BG. The influence of ethnicity and culture on the caregiver stress and coping process: A sociocultural review and analysis. Gerontologist. 1997;37(3):342-54.
3. Awadalla AW, Ohaeri JU, Al-Awadi SA, et al. Diabetes mellitus patients' family caregivers' subjective quality of life. J Natl Med Assoc. 2006;98(5):727-36.
4. Brannan AM, Heflinger CA, Bickman L. The Caregiver Strain Questionnaire: Measuring the impact on the family of living with a child with serious emotional disturbance. J Emot Behav Disord. 1997;5(4):212-22.
5. Cooke RA, Rousseau DM. Stress and strain from family roles and work-role expectations. J Appl Psychol. 1984;69(2):252-60.
6. De Berardis G, Franciosi M, Belfiglio M, et al. Erectile dysfunction and quality of life in type 2 diabetic patients. Diabetes Care. 2002;25(2):284-91.
7. Dimitraki G, Karademas EC. The association of type 2 diabetes patient and spouse illness representations with their well-being: A dyadic approach. Int J Behav Med. 2014;21(2):230-9.
8. Fisher L, Chesla CA, Skaff MM, et al. Depression and anxiety among partners of European-American and Latino patients with type 2 diabetes. Diabetes Care. 2002;25(9):1564-70.
9. Golics CJ, Basra MK, Salek MS, et al. The impact of patients' chronic disease on family quality of life: An experience from 26 specialties. Int J Gen Med. 2013;6:787-98.
10. Gonder-Frederick L, Cox D, Kovatchev B, et al. The psychosocial impact of severe hypoglycemic episodes on spouses of patients with IDDM. Diabetes Care. 1997;20(10):1543-6.
11. Holmes AM, Deb P. The effect of chronic illness on the psychological health of family members. J Ment Health Policy Econ. 2003;6(1):13-22.
12. Jaser SS, Whittemore R, Ambrosino JM, et al. Mediators of depressive symptoms in children with type 1 diabetes and their mothers. J Pediatr Psychol. 2007;33(5):509-19.
13. Kovacs M, Iyengar S, Goldston D, et al. Psychological functioning among mothers of children with insulin-dependent diabetes mellitus: A longitudinal study. J Consult Clin Psychol. 1990;58(2):189.
14. Lebrec J, Ascher-Svanum H, Chen YF, et al. Effect of diabetes on caregiver burden in an observational study of individuals with Alzheimer's disease. BMC Geriatr. 2016;16(1):93.
15. Lowes L, Lyne P, Gregory JW. Childhood diabetes: Parents' experience of home management and the first year following diagnosis. Diabet Med. 2004;21(6):531-8.
16. Montgomery RJ, Gonyea JG, Hooyman NR. Caregiving and the experience of subjective and objective burden. Family Relations. 1985:19-26.
17. Rankin ED. Caregiver stress and the elderly: A familial perspective. Journal of Gerontological Social Work. 1990;15(1-2):57-73.
18. Rhee EJ. Diabetes in Asians. Endocrinology and metabolism. 2015;30(3):263-9.
19. Sharma N, Chakrabarti S, Grover S. Gender differences in caregiving among family-caregivers of people with mental illnesses. World J Psychiatry. 2016;6(1):7-17.
20. Smaldone A, Ritholz MD. Perceptions of parenting children with type 1 diabetes diagnosed in early childhood. J Pediatric Health Care. 2011;25(2):87-95.
21. Stone R, Cafferata GL, Sangl J. Caregivers of the frail elderly: A national profile. Gerontologist. 1987;27(5):616-26.
22. Streisand R, Swift E, Wickmark T, et al. Pediatric parenting stress among parents of children with type 1 diabetes: The role of self-efficacy, responsibility, and fear. J Pediatr Psychol. 2005;30(6):513-21.
23. Whittemore R, Jaser S, Chao A, et al. Grey M. Psychological experience of parents of children with type 1 diabetes: A systematic mixed-studies review. Diabetes Educ. 2012;38(4):562-79.

27 CHAPTER

Fasts in Women with Diabetes

Sameer Aggarwal, Deep Dutta

INTRODUCTION

Fasting is defined as a partial or total abstention from all foods, or a select abstention from prohibited foods. Islamic Ramadan and Hindu Fasts have been discussed in this review. This systematic review intends to analyze all available literature for preventing glycemic excursions associated with erratic food intake coupled with prolonged fasting associated with religious festivals and provide suggestions to prevent diabetes as well as avoid diabetes complications in patients with diabetes.

The three most commonly studied fasts are:

1 Caloric restriction
2 Alternate-day fasting
3 Dietary restriction.

Caloric restriction (CR) is the reduction of kilocalorie intake by approximately 20–40% of *ad libitum* consumption. Caloric restriction appears to delay the onset of the following diseases: autoimmune diseases, atherosclerosis, cardiomyopathies, cancer, diabetes, renal diseases, neuro-degenerative diseases, and respiratory diseases. Caloric restriction improves cardiovascular health, decrease fasting glucose and insulin levels, increase insulin sensitivity, decrease body fat percentage, and lower the incidence of diabetes.

Alternate-day fasting (ADF) consists of alternating 24-hour periods: during the "feast period", fasters may consume food *ad libitum*; during the "fast period", food consumption is restricted or halted altogether. Water is allowed *ad libitum* during all times. Alternate-day fasting has beneficial changes in cardiovascular health. Regarding glucoregulatory health, ADF may have gender-specific effects. For example, ADF improved insulin sensitivity in men but had no effect on this variable in women. Furthermore, glucose tolerance was unchanged in men partaking in an ADF regimen, but women partaking in the same regimen experienced impaired glucose tolerance.

Dietary restriction (DR) is a reduction of one or more components of dietary intake (typically macronutrients) with minimal to no reduction in total kcal intake. No human data is available regarding benefits or harm of DR.

ISLAMIC FASTS

What does Fasting During Ramadan Involve?

During the month of Ramadan, Muslims abstain from either eating or drinking liquids between sunrise and sunset for 30 days. Fasting starts from early dawn *(Suhur/Sehri)* till sunset *(Iftar)*. This tends to lead to consumption of a rather large meal in the evening and a variable amount of food before dawn, which may affect glycemic control in people with diabetes.

What are the Risks of Fasting for Women with Diabetes who Fast?

The risks of fasting include hypoglycemia, hyperglycemia, and dehydration. Women at high risk for complications after fasting in diabetes are those with:

- Severe and recurrent episodes of hypoglycemia and hypoglycemic unawareness
- Those with poor glycemic control, especially those with glycosylated hemoglobin (HbA1c) >9%
- In those with ketoacidosis in the 3 months before Ramadan
- Those who experience hyperosmolar hyperglycemic coma within the 3 months before Ramadan
- Those with acute or chronic illness
- Pregnant women
- Those with comorbidities such as advanced macrovascular complications, renal disease on dialysis, cognitive dysfunction, and uncontrolled epilepsy.

Women classed as high risk are advised not to fast as it can lead to worsening diabetes control. The holy Quran exempts sick people from the duty of fasting.

How Should Fasting Women with Diabetes be Managed?

Frequent monitoring of glycemia is essential. This is especially critical in women with type 1 diabetes mellitus (T1DM) and in women with type 2 diabetes mellitus (T2DM) who require insulin.

Diet in Ramadan

Slow energy release foods (such as wheat, beans, and rice) should be taken before and after fasting, whereas foods high in saturated fat (such as ghee, samosas, and pakoras) should be minimized.

Women Taking Oral Hypoglycemic Agents

For women with T2DM taking either of dipeptidyl peptidase-4 (DPP-4) inhibitors/glucagon-like peptide-1 mimetics/thiazolidinediones, no dose adjustment is necessary. For women taking sulfonylureas once daily, switch the dose to *Iftar*. For patients taking sulfonylureas twice daily, reduce *Suhur* dose (e.g., change a twice daily dose of 80 mg gliclazide to 80 mg at *Iftar* and 40 mg at *Suhur*). For patients taking only metformin, modify timing of doses, give two-thirds of daily dose at *Iftar* and one-third of daily dose at *Suhur*. If taking modified release metformin once daily, take dose at *Iftar* rather than at *Suhur*.

Women Taking Insulin

Among women with T1DM or among insulin-requiring women with T2DM, adequate rapid-acting insulin analog for the large meal and the maintenance of basal insulin levels during the period of fasting is crucial to avoid the development of hyperglycemia and ketoacidosis.

Rapid-acting insulin analogs are helpful in both reducing the higher prandial glucose levels following the large evening meal and decreasing the likelihood of the hypoglycemia. Using carbohydrate-counting regimens for adjusting insulin doses in the calculation of meal-related boluses will help achieve optimum insulin levels.

Type-2 diabetic women on single dose of basal insulin should reduce their basal insulin dose by 20%. For patients taking twice daily insulin should reduce the *Suhur* dose by 30% if they are well-controlled, and consider switching to a mix 50 preparation if their postprandial glucose remains raised. Type 1 diabetic patients on multiple doses of insulin should reduce their basal insulin by 20% and omit the mid-day rapid-acting insulin if their capillary blood glucose concentration is less than or equal to 7 mmol/L. If their blood glucose concentration is more than 7 mmol/L, patients will need to calculate their insulin correction dose as determined by their specialists.

Pregnant women with diabetes, including gestational diabetes mellitus (GDM), are exempted from fasting and are strongly cautioned against fasting because maternal and fetal risks are associated with poor glycemic control in pregnancy. If the woman feels obliged to fast then those with GDM, controlled on medical nutrition therapy, may be allowed to fast, under close medical supervision. Women with GDM or pre-existing T2DM, well-controlled on low dose of insulin, may fast and follow insulin dose modification strategies. Women with T1DM and those with T2DM, on high or frequent dose of insulin, or with erratic/suboptimal control, must be discouraged from fasting due to the high risk for the fetus and mother. Breastfeeding women are also exempted from fasting.

HINDU FASTS

In contrast to Ramadan fasts, Hindu fasting is more varied and ranges from weekly to bi-weekly fasts to fasting extended over several days. Fasting is commonly associated with feasts, which are closely linked with different festivals overall, round the year. An extreme form of fasting is seen in Jains, where the fasting can even extend over several weeks.

Problem Issues

Fasting for prolonged periods is frequently followed by overeating and binge eating resulting in rebound hyperglycemia. Dehydration secondary to restricted fluid intake, often in the setting of stoppage of medications and insulin, increases the risk of ketoacidosis in these patients. In fact, stoppage of insulin associated with religious fasting is one of the most common causes of ketoacidosis in patients with T1DM in India. Dehydration can result in postural hypotension and syncope in patients with autonomic neuropathy along with increased risk of thrombosis and stroke secondary to hyperviscosity. Osmotic diuresis secondary to rebound hyperglycemia following overeating can result in dyselectrolytemia and altered sensorium, especially in the elderly.

Ritualistic fasting under peer and family pressure is often treated as a test of personal religious faith, often resulting in unrealistic strict abstinence from all foods; drinks, including water; and stoppage of all antidiabetic medications in patients with diabetes. Fasting during Navratri by Jains, which commonly extends beyond 24 hours and often lasts over several days, when even water is not allowed.

Which Patients Should Absolutely Avoid Fasts?

Diabetic patients with poor glycemic control (HbA1c >9%), recent history of ketoacidosis, established microvascular and macrovascular complications, severe associated comorbid states, infections, pregnancy, and those in geriatric age group, should be discouraged to undertake diet and diabetic medication modifications during festivals.

Which Patients Can Safely Fast During Festivals and Religious Events?

Stable patients of diabetes, who are willing to continue medications during Navratris and Durga pujas, motivated to do self-monitoring of blood glucose (SMBG) and with knowledge for corrective insulin boluses, aware about symptoms of hypoglycemia, hyperglycemia, osmotic symptoms, and full knowledge of diet and lifestyle interventions have the lowest risk of complications following fasting and diet changes during festivals like Holi, Deepawali, Navratris, and Durga pujas.

How to Prevent Adverse Outcomes During Fasting?

Dietary restraint is central to ensuring adequate glycemic control during festivals. One should keep a tab on number of sweets consumed. It is a good idea to consume half or even a quarter of sweet with friends and family over several sittings. Taking a smaller serving of each meal to account for increased occurrence of between meal snacking helps in keeping a tab on the calories consumed over 24 hours. Carbohydrate counting and adjusting for short-acting insulin boluses in patients on Multiple Sclerosis study II has an important role in ensuring adequate glycemic control. It is important to realize that family members and the society have an important role to play in this. The second Diabetes Attitudes Wishes and Needs (DAWN 2) study highlighted that diabetics in general across the globe feel discriminated against cause of diabetes, and especially if they are taking insulin. This is perhaps even more so in India. These feelings are accentuated during festivals.

Managing Antidiabetic Medications During Fasts

Kalra et al. have recently highlighted several issues associated with ritualistic fasting in Indian festivals, with focus on Karva Chauth, an annual day long fast kept by married Indian women in northern India, and frequent weekly fasts kept on specific days by Hindus across the country. A specific drug treatment plan focusing on Karva Chauth has been provided. The importance of prefast counseling and increasing awareness regarding hypoglycemic and hyperglycemic symptoms among patients with diabetes was also highlighted. Patients should visit their treating physician days to weeks before festival, for appropriate prefestival counseling and adjustment of their antidiabetic medications during the festival. It would be a good practice to audit the SMBG charting done by patients during festivals, for assessment of the glycemic variability so that lessons learnt can be incorporated in next year's treatment plan.

Choosing Oral Agents for Managing Fasts

Hypoglycemia risk is maximal with long-acting insulin secretagogues like sulfonylureas. Among sulfonylureas, glibenclamide has the maximum hypoglycemia risk followed by glipizide, gliclazide, and glimepiride. Patients planning for fasting greater than 12 hours duration should not take the same day or previous night sulfonylurea. Patients who plan to do prolonged intermittent fasting during Navratri and Durga pujas may be shifted from sulfonylureas to short-acting secretagogues like repaglinide or nateglinide to reduce hypoglycemia risk. Metformin, pioglitazone, α-glucosidase inhibitors, and incretin-based therapies like DPP4 inhibitors and GLP-1 analogs can be safely continued, as they have low associated risk of hypoglycemia.

How to Use Insulin in the Best Possible Way during Fasts?

Patients on premixed insulin injections twice daily may preferably be shifted to a more physiological basal bolus regimen before the onset of festival season. Premixed insulin regimens are rigid and are less equipped to handle the erratic food regimens accompanied by fasting during festivals, increasing the risk of both uncontrolled hyperglycemia and hypoglycemia. In contrast to general belief, stable patients with T1DM can fast safely up to 24 hours. In stable T1DM and T2DM patients on insulin, planning to fast for 12–24 hours, basal insulin should be continued at around 0.2 U/kg/day. Neutral Protamine Hagedorn, glargine, or detemir; either of the three long-acting insulin can be used. Premeal short-acting insulin boluses should be avoided during fasting state for obvious reasons. Self-monitoring of blood glucose is strongly recommended during the duration of fasting, at least 6 hourly, and corrective insulin boluses may be administered in case of blood glucose values exceeding 250 mg/dL. Short-acting insulin analogs (lispro, glulisine, or aspart) may be preferred over regular insulin, simply cause of their shorter duration of action as well as flexibility of administration as they can be taken immediately after food also, though evidence is lacking in this regard. Fast should be broken immediately in case of hypoglycemic symptoms and/or blood glucose values less than 70 mg/dL. The target blood glucose during fasting state is 100–200 mg/dL. It is advisable to do a home blood pressure monitoring also and adjust antihypertensive medications accordingly.

POST-FAST MEDICAL REVIEW

Post-fast, a history should be taken to enquire about biopsychosocial health and quality of life during the fasting period, and elicit subtle symptoms of hypoglycemia or hypotension. This will help plan future therapeutic strategies.

CONCLUSION

Managing diabetes in women who fast is a team-work involving the patient, family members, and treating doctor. A pre-fast consultation with the doctor can help modify the diabetes treatment regimen suitably to prevent the risk of both hypoglycemia and hyperglycemia during fasts. It is the duty of the doctor to train and educate the patient with the risks and benefits of intermittent/prolonged fasting. Support of the family members is crucial especially to limit feasting during festivals, and adjust kitchen food habits so that people with diabetes do not feel neglected. Constructive team work for fasting during festivals provides an excellent opportunity to improve the daily diet and lifestyles of an individual.

SUGGESTED READINGS

1. Al-Arouj M, Bouguerra R, Buse J, et al. Recommendations for management of diabetes during Ramadan. Diabetes Care. 2005;28:2305-11.
2. Arouj MA, Khalil SA, Buse J, et al. Recommendations for Management of Diabetes During Ramadan. Diabetes Care. 2010;33(8):1895-902.
3. Dutta D, Chowdhury S. Glycemic Emergencies: Diabetic Ketoacidosis, Hyperosmolar Nonketotic Hyperglycemia, and Hypoglycemia. In: Bajaj S (ed). ESI manual of clinical endocrinology, 2nd edition. New Delhi: Jaypee Brothers Medical Publishers (P) Ltd.; 2014. pp. 1-9.
4. Hassan A, Meo SA, Usmani AM, et al. Diabetes during Ramadan—PRE-approach model: presentation, risk stratification, education. Eur Rev Med Pharmacol Sci. 2014;18(12):1798-805.
5. Horne BD, May HT, Anderson JL, et al. Intermountain Heart Collaborative Study. Usefulness of routine periodic fasting to lower risk of coronary artery disease in patients undergoing coronary angiography. Am J Cardiol. 2008;102:814-9.
6. Hui E, Bravis V, Hassanein M, et al. Management of people with diabetes wanting to fast during Ramadan. BMJ. 2010;340:c3053.
7. Ibrahim M, Bahijri S, Tuomilehto J. Diabetes and Ramadan. Prim Care Diabetes. 2015;9(4):241-3.
8. Jaleel MA, Raza SA, Fathima NZ, et al. Ramadan and Diabetes: As-Saum (The Fasting). Indian J Endo Metab. 2011;15(4):268-73.
9. Kalra S, Bajaj S, Gupta Y, et al. Fasts, feasts and festivals in diabetes-1: Glycemic management during Hindu fasts. Indian J Endocrinol Metab. 2015;19(2):198-203.
10. Kalra S, Baruah MP. Discrimination and diabetes: Insight from the second Diabetes Attitudes Wishes and Needs (DAWN2) Study. J Soc Health Diabetes. 2015;3:56-7.
11. Kalra S, Sridhar GR, Balhara YS, et al. National recommendations: Psychosocial management of diabetes in India. Indian J Endocrinol Metab. 2013;17:376-95.
12. Kaushal K, Raina SK. "Risk approach strategy" in diabetics on fasting-evidence base through narrative review with a special focus on Ramadan fasting. J Soc Health Diabetes. 2015;3:11-5.
13. Kovacs Burns K, Nicolucci A, Holt RI, et al. Diabetes attitudes, wishes and needs second study (DAWN2TM): Cross-national benchmarking indicators for family members living with people with diabetes. Diabet Med. 2013;30:778-88.
14. Salim I, Al Suwaidi J, Ghadban W, et al. Impact of religious. Ramadan fasting on cardiovascular disease: A systematic review of the literature. Curr Med Res Opin. 2013;29:343-54.
15. Salti I, Bénard E, Detournay B, et al. EPIDIAR study group. A population-based study of diabetes and its characteristics during the fasting month of Ramadan in 13 countries: Results of the epidemiology of diabetes and Ramadan 1422/2001 (EPIDIAR) study. Diabetes Care. 2004;27:2306-11.
16. Sawhney K, Kalra B. Today's new torture culinary cruelty or dietary draconism. Int J Clin Cases Invest. 2010;1:3-4.
17. Strich D, Teomim R, Gillis D. The basal insulin dose: a lesson from prolonged fasting in young individuals with type 1 diabetes. Pediatr Diabetes. 2015;16(8):629-33.
18. Trepanowski JF, Bloomer RJ. The impact of religious fasting on human health. Nutr J. 2010;9:57.

Index

Page numbers followed by *f* refer to figure, and *t* refer to table

A

Abdomen, lateral parts of 45
Abortion, spontaneous 124
Abscess, perinephric 88
Acanthosis nigricans 50
Acarbose 31
Acne, persistent 93
Acute coronary syndrome 73
Adenosine monophosphate 110
Alcohol 132
Amenorrhea, Secondary 116
American Diabetes Association 15, 38
American Society for Reproductive Medicine 93
Amitriptyline 169
Anemia 131, 132, 135
Anorexia nervosa 116
Antenatal corticosteroid therapy 29
Antidepressants 164
Antidiabetic drugs 25
Antimitogenic activity 112
Antithyroid drugs 112
Anxiety 167
  disorders 170
Arizona sexual experience scale 162
Arousal
  disorder 160, 164, 165
Arterial hypertension, systolic 72
Atrial fibrillation 74
Auscultation, cardiac 134
Autoimmune thyroid disorders 106
Auxiliary nurse midwife 131

B

Bacteriuria, asymptomatic 87-89
Barrier methods 124, 126
Binge eating disorder 116
Birth
  control 127
  weight 16
Blood
  glucose, self-monitoring of 38, 185
  pressure 73, 132
    high 60
    measurement 135
  sugar, high 119
Body mass index 27, 93, 118, 132, 141, 144
Bone
  abnormality, management of 103
  fracture 99, 101
  health 98
  mineral density 67, 98, 99, 99*t*, 100*t*
    studies 98
Breast cancer 148
  prognosis of 154
Breastfeeding 138-142
  behavior 139
  initiation 138
  prevalence 138
Bulimia nervosa 115, 116
Bupropion 169
Burning, chronic 14

C

Calcitriol 66
Canadian Diabetes Association 38
Canagliflozin Cardiovascular Assessment Study 103
Cancer 148, 151-153, 153f
  breast 153
  colon 154
  drug therapy of 155
  endometrial 154
  laryngeal 152
  pancreatic 155
Candida albicans 90
Candida glabrata 90
Candida krusei 90
Carcinoma, endometrial 148
Cardiovascular
  disease 57, 71, 75, 78, 147
    sex-related 71

morbidity 25
mortality 25
syndromes 72*t*
Cervical caps 124
Chlamydia 133
Cholecystitis, emphysematous 88
Chronic poor metabolic control 38
Citalopram 169
Clitoral devices 164
Cognitive behavioral therapy 164, 172
Condom 124
female 124
male 124
Conjugated estrogens therapy 146
Contraception 123, 132
choices 124
emergency 124
Contraceptive
Methods
hormonal 124
nonhormonal 124
use 127*t*
Coronary
artery disease 53
heart disease 48*f*, 57, 73, 147
Cystitis, emphysematous 87, 88

D

Daily progestin oral contraceptive 124
Data of Latest National Family Health Survey 130*t*
Depomedroxyprogesterone acetate 125
Depression 167, 169
postpartum 17
Desire, disorder of 165
Desogestrel 126
Diabetes 1, 2*f*, 9, 15-17, 25, 10, 53, 57, 66, 72, 81, 82, 103, 104, 107, 108, 108*f*, 109*t*, 110, 111, 113, 127, 132, 138, 139, 144, 147, 148, 151-153, 153*f*, 158, 159*f*, 161*f*, 176-178
age- and gender-specific prevalence of 3*f*
attitudes 186
community lifestyle improvement program 22
complications of 145
control and complications trial 77, 81
drug therapy of 155
management 17, 29, 84, 103, 123, 176
mellitus 36, 14, 50, 74, 87-89, 98, 143, 167, 169, 170
gestational 2, 10, 16, 20, 29, 44, 51, 52, 58, 67, 68, 107, 110, 123, 127, 132, 135, 138, 184
type 1 5, 12, 20, 26, 36, 65, 90, 98, 99, 99*t*, 101, 101*t*, 106, 113, 115, 117*f*, 127, 139, 143, 152, 168, 177, 183
type 2 13, 19, 20, 25, 36, 44, 47, 50, 58, 66, 73, 77, 89, 92, 98, 100*t*, 101, 106, 113, 115, 118, 119, 123, 127, 138, 143, 158, 160, 177
microvascular complications of 103
neuropathy 83
pregestational 134
prevalence of 1*f*, 2
scale, appraisal of 163
self-management education 37, 38
Diabetic nephropathy, progression of 78
Diaphragms 124
Dizziness 7
Domestic violence 133
Dual-energy X-ray absorptiometry 98, 99*t*, 100*t*
Duloxetine 169
Dysglycemia 18
Dyslipidemia 53, 57, 58, 61, 72, 95, 120
clinical consequences of 59
management of 60
persisting 111
Dyspareunia 160, 164, 165
Dysthyroid optic neuropathy 108

E

Eating disorders 40, 115, 116, 117*f*, 118, 119, 119*t*
Edema 109
Endocrine Society Clinical Practice Guidelines 69
Endocrine Society Recommend Preconception Glycosylated Hemoglobin 15
End-stage renal disease 77
Enteroviruses 88
Epinephrine 25
Escherichia coli 90
Escitalopram 169
Esophageal candidiasis 88

Estradiol 106
Estrogens 49
  deficiency 61
Ethinylestradiol 126
European Society of Human Reproduction and Embryology 93

F

Family planning 135
  methods 130
  natural 124
  services, quality of 130
Fasting
  blood sugar, lower 28
  glucose 51
Female sexual functioning index 162
Ferriman-Gallaway score, modified 93
Fertility 26
  awareness 124
Fetal
  health outcomes 30
  placental transport 30
Fluoxetine 169
Fluvoxamine 169
Folic acid 133
Follicle stimulating hormone 94
Follicular epithelium 111
Foot infection 88
Fournier's gangrene 88
Fracture 31
  intervention trial 104
  rate 101
  risk assessment tool score 101
Framingham heart study 72
Fungal cystitis 88

G

Gastrointestinal
  absorption 109, 112
  infections 88
  tract 89
Genital vibrators 164
Glomerular filtration rate 78
Gluconeogenesis 29, 107, 109
Glucose 146
  6-phosphate, hepatocyte concentration of 107
  control 66
  faster absorption of 109
  homeostasis 64, 64*f*, 144
  metabolism 107
  monitoring 38
  reduced peripheral utilization of 109
  tolerance test 109
  transporter 107
Glyburide 30
  placental transport of 30
Glycemia 27
  control 29, 37, 103, 111, 169, 169*t*
Glycogenolysis 109
Goiter 108
Gonorrhea 133
Growth hormone 25, 40

H

H1N1 88
Heart 104
  and estrogen-progestin replacement study 146
  failure 72, 74
Helicobacter pylori infection 88
Hemoglobin
  glycosylated 28, 37
  high glycosylated 29
Hepatic dysfunction 29
Hepatitis 133
  B 88
  C 88
    infection 87
    virus 90
Hepatocyte 107
Hirsutism 50, 93
Hodgkin's lymphoma 152
Hormone
  luteinizing 94
  replacement therapy 59, 143, 147, 172
  therapy, postmenopausal 145
Hospital anxiety and depression scale 163, 168
Hot flashes 7
Hydramnios 29
Hyperandrogenemia
  biochemical 93
  clinical 93
Hyperglycemia 36, 38, 108, 109
  chronic 88
  management of 85
  severe 109

Hyperreflexia 135
Hypertension 53, 57, 58, 60, 61, 72, 95, 120
Hypertensive disorder 58
Hyperthyroidism 109
Hypoglycemia 5, 27, 30, 37, 87, 108, 109, 111, 140, 143, 186
  drug induced 143
  neonatal 30
  recurrent 111
  severe 120
Hyporeflexia 135
Hypothalamo-pituitary-adrenal axis 168
Hypothyroidism 108, 109

I

Infections 33, 87, 88, 133
  congenital 133
  head and neck 88
  respiratory 88
Infectious diseases, spectrum of 88
Influenza 88
Insulin 109, 155
  injection technique 44
  like growth factor binding protein 40
  neuritis 85
  reducing requirement of 111
  resistance 39
    homeostatic model assessment measurements of 144
    syndrome 61
  sensitivity 29, 65, 144
  technique questionnaire 44
  therapy 28, 37
International Association for Diabetes in Pregnancy Study Group Criteria 52
International Classification of Diseases 115
International Diabetes Federation 16, 19
Intestinal glucose absorption 29
Intramuscular implant 125
Intrauterine
  devices 124, 125, 131
    postpartum 131
  growth retardation 29
  system 125
Invasive external otitis 88
Iodothyronine deiodinase enzyme, type 2 111
Isocarboxazid 169

K

Kegel's exercises 164
Ketoacidosis 87
  diabetic 5, 36, 109, 120
Ketonuria 29
Kidney disease
  chronic 78
  diabetic 79

L

Lactate, overproduction of 107
Lactation 68
Leukocyte, polymorphonuclear 89
Levonorgestrel 125, 126
Levothyroxine replacement therapy 111
Lipid metabolism 147
Lipoprotein cholesterol
  high density 58, 72
  low-density 58, 72
Liver
  cancer 155
  infections 88
Long-acting progestin-only contraceptives methods 124
Lung auscultation 135

M

Macrosomia 29
Major histocompatibility complex 107
Medical nutrition therapy 29
Medroxyprogesterone acetate 146
Menopause 6, 17, 72, 143-145, 148
  metabolic effects of 144
Menstrual irregularities 50
Menstruation 15
Mental health 133
Metformin 29, 31, 51, 141
Mirtazapine 169
Monoamine oxidase inhibitor 169
Muscle glycogenolysis 109
Myocardial infarction 25, 58, 72, 73

N

National Health and Nutrition Examination Survey 66
National Institute for Health and Care Excellence 27, 28*t*

Necrotizing fasciitis 88
Nephropathy 14, 120, 127
  diabetic 77, 109
Neuropathy 127
  management 85
  diabetic 81, 82, 84
  peripheral 161
Noncommunicable diseases 22
Nonoral combination hormonal methods 124, 126
Norepinephrine 25
Norethindrone enanthate 125
Norgestimate 126
Nortriptyline 169
Nutrition 133

O

Obesity 47, 75
  prepregnancy 139
  reduction 22
Obstructive sleep apnea 95
Oligomenorrhea 116
Oral contraceptive
  combined 124, 126
  pills 164
    use of 2, 59
Oral estrogen delivery 146
Oral glucose tolerance test 95, 140
Oral hypoglycemic
  agents 109, 111, 141, 184
  drugs 26, 29, 31
Orgasm, disorder of 164
Orthostasis 135
Osteoporosis, treatment of 104
Ovarian cancer 154

P

Pain, knife-like 14
Pallor 109
Palpitations 108
Paroxetine 169
Pelvic exercises 164
Peroxisome proliferator-activated receptor 64
Pharmacologic therapy 165
Phenelzine 169
Phosphodiesterase 5 inhibitors 164
Polycystic ovary
  morphology 93
  syndrome 2, 13, 26, 51, 92, 93, 95, 96, 107, 110
    management of 96
    metabolic effects of 94
Polyglandular autoimmune syndrome 107
Postmenopausal estrogen-progestin interventions 59, 144
Preeclampsia 16
Pregnancy 10, 16, 27, 68, 127
Premature death 120
Progesterone 106
Progestin only contraceptives 124
Progestogens 146
Proteinuria 78
Psychosexual therapy 164
Puberty 39, 50
Pyelonephritis, emphysematous 87

Q

Quantitative computed tomography 101

R

Relaxation therapy 164
Renal dysfunction 29
Renin-angiotensin-aldosterone system 64, 65
Retinopathy 120, 127
Rhinocerebral mucormycosis 88

S

Serotonin reuptake inhibitors 172
Sertraline 169
Serum total testosterone 93
Sexual
  desire, disorder of 160, 164
  dysfunction 160
    etiopathogenesis of 161*f*
    female 17
  health 7, 158
  response cycle 159, 159*f*
Sexually transmitted infections 133, 136
Sick-euthyroid syndrome 108
Skin 88
Sodium-glucose cotransporter 85
Soft tissue infections 88
Spermicides 124
Streptococcus pneumoniae 88
Stress 2, 134
  oxidative 111

Stroke 147
Sweating 7, 108, 109
Sympathetic nervous system 168
Syphilis 133

T

Tachycardia 109
Testosterone 164
Tetracyclic antidepressants 169
Thiazolidinediones 103, 155
Thiazolidione 32
Thyoxine 106, 109
Thyroid 107, 113, 134
  antibodies 111
  cancer 11, 110, 112
  diabetes 109
  disorders 106, 111, 113
    management of 111
    prevalence of 108f
    spectrum of 108
  dysfunction 108, 109t
    metformin-induced 112
  gland 110
  health 106
  hormone 106, 107
    metabolism 112
    protein binding 112
  nodule
    development 108
    size 112
  peroxidase 113
  physiology 108
  receptors 112
  stimulating hormone 110, 112, 113
    level, metformin reduces 109
    level, mild elevated 111
Transdermal
  estrogen delivery 146
  patch 126
Tranylcypromine 169
Tricyclic antidepressants 172
Triglycerides 72
Triiodothyronine 106, 109
Tuberculosis 88

U

United Kingdom Prospective Diabetes Study 84
United States Renal Data System 78
Unrecognized diabetic neuropathic syndrome 84
Urinary tract infection 14, 87-89
  recurrent 14

V

Vaginal
  delivery 142
  dilatation 164, 165
  ring 126
Venlafaxine 169
Vitamin D 63-67, 68*t*, 134
  deficiency 63, 67, 111
    correction of 69
    management of 68
    treatment of 69t
  promotes pancreatic beta-cell function 64
  receptor 63, 67
  regulates calcium metabolism 63
  role of 64*f*
  supplementation 65-68
Vulval pain syndrome 14
Vulvodynia 14, 84
  diabetic 14, 15
Vulvovaginal
  candidiasis 90
  infection 90
Vulvovaginitis 87

W

Waist-hip ratio 26
World health organization recommendations 136

Y

Yoga 164